Brief Psychological In
in Clinical Practice

612 WIL

DATE DUE

29/3/10			

Brief Psychological Interventions in Clinical Practice

Ann Williamson **MB ChB BSCAH Accred**
General Practitioner and Therapist

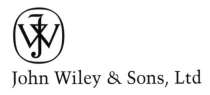

John Wiley & Sons, Ltd

Other Wiley Editorial Offices

John Wiley & Sons Inc., 111 River Street, Hoboken, NJ 07030, USA

Jossey-Bass, 989 Market Street, San Francisco, CA 94103-1741, USA

Wiley-VCH Verlag GmbH, Boschstr. 12, D-69469 Weinheim, Germany

John Wiley & Sons Australia Ltd, 42 McDougall Street, Milton, Queensland 4064, Australia

John Wiley & Sons (Asia) Pte Ltd, 2 Clementi Loop #02-01, Jin Xing Distripark, Singapore
129809

John Wiley & Sons Canada Ltd, 6045 Freemont Blvd, Mississauga, ONT, L5R 4J3, Canada

Wiley also publishes its books in a variety of electronic formats. Some content that appears in
print may not be available in electronic books.

Library of Congress Cataloging-in-Publication Data

Williamson, Ann, Dr.
   Brief psychological interventions in practice / Ann Williamson.
      p.   ;   cm.
   Includes bibliographical references and index.
      ISBN 978-0-470-51306-4 (pbk. : alk. paper)   1. Brief psychotherapy.   I. Title.
      [DNLM: 1. Psychotherapy, Brief–methods.   2. Behavioral Medicine–methods.   3. Mental
Disorders–therapy.   4. Professional-Patient Relations.   5. Psychophysiologic Disorders–therapy.
WM 420.5.P5 W729b 2008]
   RC480.55.W55 2008
   616.89′14–dc22
                                                                                    2008002746

British Library Cataloguing in Publication Data

A catalogue record for this book is available from the British Library

ISBN 978-0-470-51306-4 (pbk)

Typeset in 10 on 13 pt Scala by SNP Best-set Typesetter Ltd., Hong Kong
Printed and bound in Great Britain by TJ International Ltd, Padstow, Cornwall

Contents

About the Author

Having obtained her medical degree at Bristol University in 1972, Ann Williamson (www.annwilliamson.co.uk) became a General Practitioner in 1974. She trained in the use of hypnosis in 1989 and gained Accreditation by the British Society of Medical & Dental Hypnosis in 1995. She also trained in Neuro-linguistic Programming (NLP), becoming a Certified Practitioner in NLP in 1997 and a Master Practitioner in 1998. She has also attended many other courses and workshops on other psychological approaches including Brief Therapy presented by Bill O'Hanlon, Danie Beaulieu and Steve De Shazer.

She has been involved for over fifteen years with running training courses on hypnosis for health professionals for the Lancashire and Cheshire branch of the British Society of Medical & Dental Hypnosis and for the British Society of Experimental and Clinical Hypnosis, who now form the British Society of Clinical & Academic Hypnosis (www.bscah.co.uk). She has also run courses on hypnosis and stress management for the Postgraduate Dental Departments of Cardiff, Preston, Liverpool and North Wales among others.

Although now retired from General Practice she continues to do 2–3 hours of psychotherapy facilitated by hypnosis each week. This latter involves helping clients with unresolved grief, past traumatic experiences, post traumatic stress syndrome and phobias such as needle phobia, flying phobia etc. She has also used hypnosis with obstetric clients for pain relief and in panic disorder.

She has run Stress Management and Personal Development courses in Canada and the UK together with workshops on brief psychological interventions in Oldham, Taunton, Bury and at the European Conferences of Hypnosis in Munich and Rome.

Over the last few years Ann Williamson has also been running workshops that she calls 'Creative Wellbeing' which combine stress management and the expressive arts.

She has always been interested in why people react so differently to similar events and how people maintain problem emotional states. Increasingly frustrated with the poor and underfunded mental health service and, along with many of her patients, disinclined to use medication alone to help with emotional problems, she became interested in brief effective approaches that she could use to help her patients help themselves.

Introduction

▶ The background

The most common mental health problems are, as you might expect, anxiety and depression; panic disorder is less common but very disabling to those that suffer from it. Everyone experiences difficulties in life from time to time but, as I will show later, many people feel unable to access skills that would enable them to face life with a greater degree of resilience. When they start to feel anxious or depressed, they often consult a health professional and expect 'treatment'. I hope to show that this 'medicalisation' of feelings is counterproductive and breeds dependency rather than self-reliance.

Anxiety and depression often go hand in hand, with one aspect merely becoming more prominent at different times. Indeed, I would maintain that I have rarely, if ever, seen a client with symptoms solely attributable to anxiety or to depression alone.

Many people with anxiety begin to show agoraphobic symptoms as they draw their boundaries closer and closer in. Physical symptoms are produced by emotional distress and are often the presenting complaint. Many other conditions are made worse by low mood and anxiety; most notably conditions with chronic pain; psychosomatic disorders such as irritable bowel syndrome, migraine, excema, fibromyalgia, chronic fatigue syndrome and obsessive–compulsive disorder. Low mood and anxiety also play a part in poor compliance with treatment in conditions such as heart disease, asthma and diabetes.

I have worked in a semi-rural general practice for more than 30 years and during this time, I have seen an increasing number of people presenting with stress-related symptoms and depression. Recently, I have reckoned that more than a third of the people that I have seen in my GP surgery have a significant degree of emotional distress, be it anxiety, depression or anger.

▶ Prevalence of the problem

There have been various surveys carried out nationally that have put the incidence of 'neurotic' disorders between one in six (Office of National Statistics, 2000) and one in four adults (Goldberg & Huxley, 1992) at any one time. The term 'neurotic' covers a range of different symptoms and the different figures found in these surveys depend on what criteria have been used.

These figures contrast with that given for the incidence of psychosis and schizophrenia, which is about 1 in 200 adults at any one time. Despite this, our current mental health services are geared mainly towards helping this severe end of the spectrum. GPs and other health professionals have to try and help the vast majority of those presenting with mental health problems with little, if any. help from their local mental health teams.

Out of 1,000 people, there will be 300 or so experiencing mental health issues. Of these, 230 will visit their GP but only 102 will be diagnosed as having mental health problems. The remainder will perhaps not be given a diagnostic label as such but will still have symptoms of distress. Of those 102 diagnosed, only 24 will be referred to mental health services and 6 of these will end up as in-clients. (Goldberg & Huxley, 1992). So the vast majority of people who present with emotional distress of one kind or another are not offered help by our current system of care.

These surveys, of course, do not take into account the large number of people who present with physical symptoms allied to emotional distress; either because they feel more comfortable presenting with a physical rather than an emotional problem or because they somatise their distress without being aware that they are so doing.

The figures above were procured in 1992 but trends generally would indicate that far from the problem easing, it is getting worse, and figures for 2006 are likely to be higher again than those found in the survey done in 2000, which itself was higher than the earlier study. The numbers involved and the emotional distress implied by these figures is alarming and yet what is mainstream medicine doing effectively to combat it?

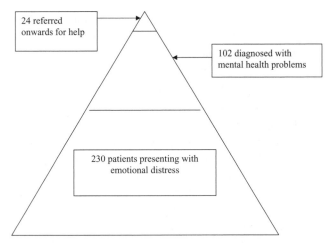

Figure i.1 Representation of the proportions of those diagnosed and referred onwards following a presentation of mental health issues

▶ The biopsychosocial perspective

Does this increase mean that people are coping less well or that life has simply become more stressful? I think both apply. Roles have changed over the years, expectations have grown, the ethos of profit before everything has taken root, certainly within most businesses; often at the expense of the ethos of caring. Employees are expected to give 110%, are forced by circumstances to work long hours and often feel undervalued and unappreciated. Working at this pitch means there is no slack in the system and when someone falls ill with stress, further strain is placed on those remaining. People feel time-pressured and often feel guilty or begrudge the time to enjoy themselves. Very often, the first thing someone does as they feel pressured or stressed is to stop going regularly to the gym, running or swimming, just at a time when they need such activities most. It is now the norm for both parents to be working, often full-time, and so trying to juggle work and child care is now a very common stressful situation.

Employees will also suffer a period of time before they actually go off sick when they are not working efficiently. Because they are stressed, they will make more mistakes, lack concentration and not be giving of their best. All this as well as the direct cost to industry of working days lost through stress, anxiety and depression, which is reckoned to be around 60 million working days (Sainsburg Centre for Mental Health, 2004). The cost of work-related mental health problems is reckoned to be around £23.1 billion pounds a year. In 2005, a survey found that one in five adults experienced their job as 'very' or 'extremely' stressful (Health and Safety Executive, 2005). Employees are the most important part of any company and yet are often the least regarded.

Whereas once people had repetitive mundane physical tasks to perform, now there are machines 'to make life easier'. We no longer have time to walk from 'A' to 'B' but have to jump in the car and sit cursing in traffic jams. The extra leisure time that all our labour-saving devices were supposed to engender has failed to materialise. We feel guilty if we sit quietly 'being' rather than 'doing'; we mustn't 'waste time'! The pace of life is so fast and, for many of us, there are so many balls to juggle, that it seems difficult to do anything else. Slumped watching television in the evening does not help us to remain mentally and emotionally healthy.

The extended family of years gone by, with all its faults, had an important supportive role to play and now rarely functions in such a way. The rising tides of marital break-up and relationship problems are sowing seeds of future problems within the next generation. Many people feel isolated and unsupported.

The messages that the media and our current culture give the young are those of the importance of instant gratification and the feeling that such gratification is theirs by right. The downside of the welfare state seems to be that people are taking less and less responsibility for themselves; whether it be for their actions or for their emotional state. The culture of litigation, of trying to find something or someone to blame, preferably to provide monetary recompense, does little to foster self-reliance and self-responsibility.

▶ To treat or not to treat?

The health professions' energies have been directed at helping those with 'enduring' and severe mental illness and this is fine so long as we bear in mind that we also need to help those with less severe problems. Their suffering should not be viewed as trivial and can often be prolonged. A follow-up survey in 2001 (Office of National Statistics, 2001) showed that half the people reported as suffering from neurotic disorders had not recovered 18 months later. Those who had received treatment were twice as likely to have recovered in this time. So intervention is useful. The question is what intervention should one use?

There seems to be an increasing tendency for us to medicalise feelings. If someone is unhappy and sinks into depression, we view it as an illness, an imbalance of chemicals within the brain. We prescribe medication, the depression lifts and another satisfactory statistic is born. But if nothing else changes, if the person concerned does not develop a different way of coping or being in the world, then relapse is probable. This is not to say that medication does not have a role to play. When someone is too distressed to be able to take any action to help themselves, then medication can certainly help to give them some internal strength to begin to do things differently. But chemical imbalance is only a small part of the story. When certain chemicals are found to be raised or lowered in anxiety and depression, how can we say that this is cause and effect, rather than merely correlation? The research supporting biochemical imbalances is rudimentary and unconvincing. Valstein (1998) suggests that psychotropic drugs create rather than cure biochemical problems because of the brain's plasticity and ability to rapidly adapt to pharmaceutical substances.

Surveys confirm that mental health problems are affected by a person's circumstances as well as by their personality. Each person lives within a context and cannot be taken in isolation from their surroundings. The social aspects of mental health problems are fairly obvious to most. Poor housing, financial difficulties, lack of family support, relationship breakdown and work stress must all contribute to the emotional distress suffered by someone with mental health problems of anxiety and depression. 'Illnesses do not just reside in organs and individuals, they are also relational and contextual' (Asen et al., 2004).

Personal resilience is, of course, hugely important as a factor in helping someone overcome such difficulties. Someone who has poor self-esteem or who has developed a negative view of the world because of a past history of physical, emotional or sexual abuse will be more prone to develop anxiety and depression.

But are our personalities set in stone? We may have a genetic predisposition to certain ways of behaving and feeling, but we can change our beliefs about ourselves and begin to learn different ways of being. Many clients come into the consulting room and tell me that they are 'born worriers'. Our job is to lead them to see that they have *learnt* how to worry, that they have a choice and that they can learn other ways of behaving and feeling. Someone may have a family history of depression and have learnt ways of responding to life that ends up with their having recurrent bouts of depression but they can relearn a more resourceful way of responding that can turn their life around.

▶ Medication – the way forward?

Because health professionals, especially GPs, have only a limited consultation time with those suffering anxiety and depression the help offered is usually medication; with maybe a suggestion to go and see a counsellor. Every time we write a prescription, we start to build a dependency upon the doctor or health professional. Between 1992 and 2000, the number of people receiving medication for anxiety and depression had doubled, whereas the number receiving psychological help remained level.

The total cost of antidepressant prescribing in 2004 was over £400 million (Office of National Statistics, 2005). Selective serotonin reuptake inhibitors (SSRIs) account for more than half of this and are now prescribed for anxiety as well as depression (Prescription Pricing Authority, 2005). Prescribing of these has rocketed by around 45% over the last five years. The costs to the UK National Health Service (NHS) are alarming, with no end in sight.

Apart from the enormous costs of these drugs, are they actually effective?

It is very probable that side effects may account for the effects seen in antidepressant studies – a review of the 13 studies available in 1994 showed positive correlation between side effects and improvement (Greenberg et al., 1994). Meta-analysis of 19 studies (2,318 clients) showed 75% of the beneficial effect can be ascribed to placebo effect . . . the remaining 25% to the side effects. When an active placebo is used the advantage of the antidepressant disappears (Kirsch & Sapirstein, 1998). Other studies support the placebo counting for most of the antidepressant effect (Joffe, Sokolov & Streiner, 1996). In my own experience, clients may start medication and then stop it after a couple of days because of side effects but actually start to improve, which certainly cannot be because of the drug as it would not have had sufficient intake to be effective. It is as though they have been 'kick-started' into feeling better; maybe it is that they realise they feel so much worse with the medication that when they stop, the feelings of relative well-being start to generate a more positive feedback loop.

Another meta-analysis of 22 antidepressant studies with 2,230 clients in 1992 showed that both old and new antidepressants showed about 20% advantage over placebo on clinician-rated measures but none on client-rated measures (Greenberg et al., 1992).

This highlights another important point. The client is the most important factor and their subjective feelings is what determines their reality – not the clinician's rating on a scale.

In the Treatment of Depression Collaborative Research Project, 250 clients were assigned randomly to cognitive therapy, interpersonal therapy, antidepressant treatment and placebo. All four had similar success in outcome measures at the end of the trial (Elkin *et al.*, 1989) but on an 18-month follow-up, psychotherapies outperformed medication and placebo on nearly every outcome measure (Shea *et al.*, 1992).

Meta-analysis of seven well-controlled studies of 513 clients concluded that of 100 clients with major depression, 29 would recover on medication alone, 47 on therapy alone and 47 with combined approach; dropout or poor response can be expected on 52 drug clients, 30 therapy clients and 34 combined clients (Wexler & Cicchetti, 1992).

A widely cited study supporting use of anti-anxiety drugs showed total cure of panic attacks after four weeks – significantly more than for placebo (Klerman, 1988). But if you look at the data for eight weeks, any advantage over placebo has disappeared and after eight weeks, the number of panic attacks were greater than at treatment entry (Danton & Antonuccio, 1997).

▶ What are the alternatives?

Over the years, I have begun to realise that many people *do* want to help themselves, if only they knew how. There are many that do not want to take medication for their depression, anxiety or panic attacks. They want to learn ways to help themselves. One of the roles of health professionals is to help people to do just that. How can we begin to do that, given the time constraints most of us work under? Hopefully, this book will begin to answer that question.

The counselling and psychotherapy professions have sprung up like mushrooms to try and help people cope with their feelings and often do a good job. But, and it is a big but, what do we do with people who can't afford or who have no access to long-term psychotherapy or counselling?

Not all health professionals have an interest in mental health but some of the interventions that I wish to explore in this book are so simple that anyone can use them. It does not need a great shift in the way one works; it is more the change in one's way of thinking that is important. We have a duty of care to our clients that I do not feel we fulfil if we do not learn the skills needed to give people the tools they need to help themselves. I want to help create the expectancy that clients can help themselves. It is so much more satisfying to work with clients towards the goals they set themselves even though it takes more effort initially, for both them and us, than prescribing medication.

The World Health Organisation definition of health is that of 'a state of complete physical, mental and social well-being, not merely the absence of disease or infirmity'. I was at a conference a year or two ago where I heard an eminent professor declare that this definition was ridiculous, as it was impossible to attain. But we get what we focus on, and if we can help even a few individuals to progress towards that goal, then it is worth going for.

CHAPTER ONE

GP or therapist – or both?

> The medical model, emphasising diagnostic classification and cures, has been transplanted wholesale into the field of human problems (Duncan & Miller, 2000, p. 19).

The western medical model

Our western medical model is based upon assessing the problem, making a diagnosis and then prescribing the correct treatment. Neat, tidy and easily quantifiable! The problem is that when we try and match this across to mental health issues, we immediately run into difficulties. We are dealing with complex human beings with a myriad of ideas, beliefs, expectations and symptoms that rarely fit snugly into a single label.

Primary care practitioners have been brought up and trained in the medical model and often feel most comfortable when working in this way. But what are we doing to our clients? If you medicalise a condition, whether anxiety, depression or addiction, you imply that the cause is probably inbuilt or genetic, that the client is relatively powerless to change and that the doctor will provide a 'cure' or 'manage' the condition. This may be good for the professional's ego but does little to teach the client new perspectives or new skills.

Pathologising emotions

We continually talk about emotional distress as an illness or pathology that needs to be 'cured'. Perceived wisdom is that if you are mildly depressed then counselling may help, whereas moderate to severe depression requires medication. But it has been shown that there is no relationship between diagnosis, selection of approach and outcome (Beutler, 1998; Beutler & Clarkin, 1990). How can you be 'mildly' depressed? You can be unhappy, fed up, pissed off, depressed but each label has a spread of attributes and is multifactorial.

We need to learn how to deal with adversity in a resourceful way – it is unrealistic to think that we will feel happy all the time. Positive thinking may help but only up to a point! We need to teach our clients how to begin to tolerate uncertainty, to tolerate sometimes feeling low or anxious in the knowledge that they can learn the skills they need to keep emotionally healthy if they do not have them already.

Unfortunately, Health Professionals, especially GPs, have huge time constraints and often it seems much more time-effective to reach for the prescription pad than expend time and energy on other approaches.

The health professional may have worries that leaving the security of their standard approach may take too much time or cause them to expend too much energy. The ideas presented in this book are not rocket science but like most effective things, quite simple. It depends more on a change in mindset of the health professional than any deep and profound additional knowledge.

▶ The first steps

Coming to see a health professional can in itself be therapeutic; after all, the word therapy comes from the Greek word for 'attendance'. How the health professional directs the consultation will dictate whether it is therapeutic or not.

I have found that asking the right question, noticing the minimal cues that the client gives me and listening to what the client is actually saying cuts consultation time down because the client begins to focus on their strengths and we cut to the heart of the problem and the solution much more quickly. Very often, if you do not pick up on something the client has said, maybe not noticed some non-verbal feedback, then the whole consultation is spent barking up the wrong tree and getting nowhere.

▶ Applicability of the medical model

There are times when one very definitely needs the medical model – one needs to exclude pathology when dealing with pain, one needs to treat the heart failure or diabetes. If someone has a heart attack, one needs to act quickly within the medical model. But one needs to be aware, once the medical emergency is over, that the client has emotional issues that need addressing. I have met several people who had previously been very fit and well, who, following a sudden heart attack become depressed and overly worried about their physical symptoms. They become cardiac invalids, even when there is, from a medical viewpoint, nothing to stop them leading a normal life.

I believe that good and effective GPs already, very often, act as therapists. Some, dependant upon character, inclination or training will feel uncomfortable in this role, but using the techniques outlined in this book will make it easier for them to deliver drip-feed psychotherapy to those clients who are willing and eager to learn new skills or re-awaken old ones.

▶ Problems with being a therapist

Health professionals also need a degree of realism. Most people can be helped; some greatly, some only in minor ways, but health professionals are not going to be able to help everyone all the time. The Messiah complex, the feeling that you can help everyone, is not only unrealistic, it is unhealthy. It is important that anyone who is trying to help people with emotional issues should ensure that they pay attention to their own emotional health. If we are feeling tired, low in mood or stressed, we cannot give our best to our clients and everything seems an uphill struggle. Maybe we should use for ourselves some of the ideas in this book before we teach our clients, in order to stay emotionally healthy ourselves.

One difference between primary care clinicians and therapists is that most therapists work with supervision and have someone with whom they can share the highs and lows of therapy. GPs tend not to have this, but if it is at all possible it is very useful to meet a colleague and discuss cases, even if it is only over coffee! Sharing one's thoughts about a case not only elicits support and reassurance from a peer but can also stimulate creative therapeutic ideas.

Classically, the health professional feels tired and dispirited after having had a consultation with a 'heartsink' client. With the approaches described in this book, because there is some structure and the client feels validated and listened to, the health professional's energy levels are not sapped by focusing on the client's problems. Taking a psychological perspective in such cases has been shown to be useful (Balint, 1957; Elder & Holmes, 2002).

It is important to step into a client's shoes so as to begin to understand them, but it is important to keep our own shoes on as well. If we become immersed in a client's problem then there are two people with a difficulty rather than one. Equally, it is unwise to take the 'expert' role as this disempowers the client and buys into the medicalisation of emotional distress. I like the concept of being a 'travelling companion rather than a travel agent' (Deitchman, 1980, p. 789).

One of the fears that I think many primary care physicians have is that they will get swamped by clients if they start to work with their emotional problems. In my experience, if you structure it correctly then those 'heartsink' or 'fat file' clients whom you work with will actually start to rely on you less and eventually see you much less frequently, as well as using up less resources with investigations and medication. Also, because we are both focused on, and working towards, the same goal, it stops that sinking feeling that we may often feel when Mrs Bloggs comes in again for the second time that week with a myriad of different symptoms, none of which fit neatly into a diagnostic label and which leave the doctor feeling confused and frustrated.

▶ Setting the contract

Deciding with the client on what their goal or goals are and together defining how often and for how long you should meet is essential, especially for clients with great emotional needs. A regular review of progress is also essential and can alert you to problems that are blocking progress. These can then be explored. We will talk more about goal setting in later chapters but deciding on these parameters right at the start and allowing the client to tell you how often they think they should see you and 'negotiating' a plan means that the client 'owns' this decision.

The other advantage of the client 'owning' the decision as to when to come for a consultation means that less time is wasted on DNAs (did not attend).

Case 1: David

David was a 57-year-old mechanic who had been out of work for two years with stress and depression. He comes to the surgery frequently with various physical complaints and symptoms and has been on an antidepressant for several months with no noticeable improvement.

After explanation, he is keen to try a different approach and we decide to have a 10-minute consultation every week for one month and review progress.

At the month review, there has been a noticeable improvement and when asked how often he needs to attend surgery now, David suggests every two weeks.

We decide to meet every two weeks for two months and review.

By eight weeks, he is doing so well that we lengthen the time between consultations to four weeks . . .

▶ **Selection**

Some clients do not wish to work with you on their emotional problems. They want the doctor to take control and give them something that will 'make them better'. Sometimes one can gradually lead such people to take a different perspective but there are many clients who are willing and eager to start to take control of their lives, so perhaps we should look at where we can most usefully direct our energies and be a little selective as to whom we should take on for formal therapy. The ideas in this book can, however, inform all of your consultations and be implemented less formally when appropriate. Try taking a solution-oriented, rather than a problem-focused, stance generally and notice how your consultations change. . . .

There are times when it is not appropriate to begin working with someone on their difficulties, but there are still tools that you can teach that are simple and effective.

When someone is drowning, it is not the time to offer them a swimming lesson – but one can throw them a lifebelt.

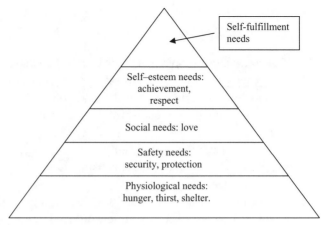

Figure 1.1   Maslow's hierarchy of needs

Sometimes the health professional needs to decide whether support or change is appropriate in a particular case. Sometimes practical help is needed before any emotional difficulties can be addressed. Maslow's hierarchy comes to mind: when someone is worrying about where their next meal is coming from or where they can stay because they are homeless, it seems inappropriate to focus attention on their emotional state. They have pressing practical needs that have to be addressed first.

▶ Onward referral

This book deals with ways of helping people with anxiety and depression, with the common neurotic disorders that we all suffer with from time to time. The severe end of the spectrum of mental illness (I'm afraid going back to the medical model here) such as psychosis needs onward referral to specialist services in the acute stage. But once settled, a solution-focused approach is eminently suitable and learning some of the ways described in this book to break into previous patterns of behaviour can be useful and effective.

When working with people at the high-risk end of the spectrum, those that are likely to self-harm or harm others, it is of great importance that the health professional does not work in isolation and that they work within their field of expertise and training. Alerting the local mental health team so that support can be given and keeping good notes are essential.

▶ Disengagement

Disengagement is less of a problem when working in the way I describe because the approach is collaborative and the focus is on helping the clients help themselves. Sometimes it is necessary to disengage slowly and to build a client's confidence that they can manage without your support by gradually lengthening the time between consultations. Primary care physicians are in an especially good position to keep minimal support for clients when appropriate, by seeing them for a follow-up appointment every few months, for a while.

I find asking the client to decide when they next need to see you can be very helpful. It gives the client confidence and control and if the health professional feels that the time selected is not appropriate, it can be a useful pointer to further work required and can be subject to negotiation.

With some clients, particularly those with a borderline personality disorder, it is necessary to define with the client, at the outset, a contract that you yourself are comfortable with.

This is where review can be so useful; if progress is not being made towards the client's goals, then it is necessary to disengage or try something different. Two quotes seem appropriate here:

> When you discover you're riding a dead horse, the best strategy is to dismount.
>
> Native American Dakota tribal wisdom

> It is common sense to take a method and try it. If it fails, admit it frankly and try another.
> But above all, try something.
>
> Franklin D. Roosevelt

▶ Relapse

It is commonly found that clients improve during the therapeutic process, but then relapse after disengagement. Using the methods described in the following chapters, relapse is considered and strategies devised with the client that minimises this risk, although sometimes clients need to return for a few 'refresher' consultations. As health professionals, we can work for a while with clients until they reach a stage that is satisfactory for them and then, if a crisis arises, see them again for a while, until things stabilise or improve.

Recovery does not mean that a person will no longer experience symptoms; it is much more about how they live their life in the midst of those symptoms. We all face setbacks and find life a struggle at times and should take care not to blur the margins between these and a person's symptoms. We must 'stop pathologising daily life and focus instead on how we can better navigate through life's difficulties to help people achieve what they desire' (Rapp & Goscha, 2006).

▶ Time constraints

We work under huge time constraints but all the ideas presented in the following chapters I have used successfully within 10-minute consultations. Sometimes it is necessary to schedule a double appointment time, but in my experience once the health professional starts working from the perspectives suggested in this book, the time is just used in a much more effective and focused way.

It is entirely possible to use these tools within groups, and over the years, I have run many groups of 6 to 10 clients where we work to these ideas over two-to-three-hour sessions and then offer individual sessions if needed later.

▶ Summary

If alcoholism, depression or smoking is regarded as an 'illness', it then follows that:

1. It is not my fault.

2. I can do nothing about it.

3. I take tablets to correct the problem.

4. It is genetic.

5. The doctor is powerful.

6. The patient is powerless.

However, one needs to exclude pathology especially when dealing with physical symptoms, such as pain, but equally the health professional needs to address emotional issues when dealing with physical pathology.

We, as health professionals, need to have regard to our own emotional well-being and this should involve someone to talk to about difficult issues that may arise. Do not try and be a Messiah – you can help many clients – but only those that want to be helped. Utilise a solution-focused approach and be aware of when onward referral is appropriate. Always work within your field of clinical expertise and keep reasonable notes and you are unlikely to find yourself in trouble.

Set a contract with your client both as regards frequency of contact and the goals you are working towards. Disengagement is not a problem if you regularly monitor progress towards these goals.

CHAPTER TWO

Problem- or solution-based?

▶ The historical perspective

Psychology as a science developed gradually from the natural sciences and philosophies into the psychoanalytical approach at the beginning of the twentieth century (Boeree, 2000). Empirical methods used in natural sciences led emerging professions to define themselves as sciences rather than as crafts or philanthropic pursuits. The focus became less on improving the moral fibre of the less fortunate and mentally ill but more towards the development of logical and rational theoretical structures and treatment (Rapp & Goscha, 2006). This led to psychology developing a pathology of negative emotional states, reified in the *Diagnostic and Statistical Manual of Mental Disorders* (DSM IV), the clinical diagnostic categories and labels given to mental illness. There is a belief that until a cause or condition has been diagnosed, a treatment cannot be successful; that there is a strong relationship between defining the problem, identifying the cause and solving the problem. This is appropriate when dealing with machines but unfortunately human beings and their problems are rather more complex. The very term 'treatment' implies a problem orientation and denotes the dual role of client and doctor/therapist.

▶ Psychological ideas in the twentieth century

Freud developed ideas of the unconscious, the model of the id, ego and superego, and the premise that all behaviour and symptoms develop because of 'repressed' material in the unconscious which has to be made 'conscious' for the symptom to be resolved (Alexander,

1946; Winnicott, 1958). From the 1930s onwards, there was increasing interest in psychoanalytic theory as a theoretical framework for defining people's problems. This, of course, meant that the focus of assessment, diagnosis and treatment was placed firmly on the problems or deficits of the client.

Therapy had no obvious end point or outcome measurements and was therefore often extremely prolonged and only affordable by the wealthy.

Over the twentieth century, many different psychological therapies developed, directly stemming from a reaction against the psychoanalytical model.

Jung and Adler started out with Freud's model but then developed other ideas, which led towards other more psychodynamic approaches in psychotherapy. Alfred Adler's Individual Psychology was a forerunner of modern cognitive therapies with the theory that one's opinions and beliefs are the primary determinants of behaviour (Ellis, 1973, 1989; Murray & Jacobson, 1978).

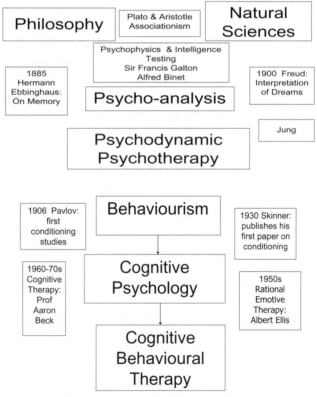

Figure 2.1 Psychology – evolution of different models

But psychodynamic theories were also problem-based in the belief that the emotional sequelae and reactions to events in a person's past past were causative and underpinned that persons' current psychological problems. Treatment is focused on resolving the difficulty in the past so as to lessen its negative emotional impact on the present.

Ideas about conditioning (Wolpe, 1958) developed into behaviourism, where changing the behaviour manifested by the client was the focus of therapy rather than the exploration of its causes (Eysenk, 1976; Skinner, 1953). Although ideas that cognition could play a major role in client's problems had been around earlier in the twentieth century, it was not until the 1950s that Albert Ellis developed Rational Emotive Therapy (Ellis, 1962) and later still Professor Aaron Beck started to develop cognitive psychology. Cognitive behavioural therapy (CBT) developed from both these approaches and is popular today. CBT also focuses on conscious thoughts, known as 'automatic thoughts' (Beck, 1976) or 'internal dialogue' (Meichenbaum, 1977) that reflect peoples' beliefs and ideas, that in turn drive their emotional responses or behaviour.

Carl Rodgers was influential in bringing a humanistic client-centred approach into therapy in the 1950s, that underpins most of the counselling used today. Gestalt and other humanistic therapies also arose from these ideas.

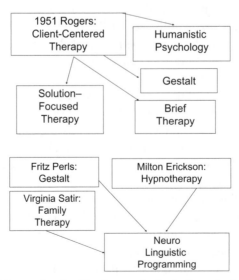

Figure 2.2   Schema showing development of solution-oriented approaches.

'Approaches differ in the way the problem is defined, but virtually all schools of therapeutic thought maintain the belief that people need help because they have a problem . . . that in some way sets them apart from people who are thought not to have that problem' (Rapp & Goscha, 2006). This of course is a nice rationale for professional helpers.

▶ New ideas

In the 1970s, Richard Bandler (a mathematician) and John Grinder (a linguist) decided to study the most successful therapists of the time. Those they selected were Milton H. Erickson, MD, widely regarded as the founder of modern hypnotherapy; Fritz Perls, founder of gestalt therapy; and Virginia Satir, a family therapist. They studied their interactions and interventions made in the therapeutic sessions with their clients and broke these down into their component parts. Gradually, they developed a way of understanding how people build their subjective reality and how they initiate and maintain behaviours (Andreas & Andreas, 1987; Bandler & Grinder, 1981). This was then marketed as neuro-linguistic programming (NLP) and used widely in the advertising business as well as in psychotherapy (McDermott & O'Connor, 1996).

At around the same time, brief and solution-focused therapy (S de Shazer, 2005; Shazer, 1988; Shazer *et al.*, 1986) were being pioneered in the States as a direct backlash to the lengthy psychoanalytical approaches mainly used at the time. Steve de Shazer and his wife Insoo Kim Berg and their team at the Brief Family Therapy Family Center in Milwaukee, USA were working in the early 1980s building on the work of a number of other innovators, among them Milton Erickson, and the group at the Mental Research Institute at Palo Alto – Gregory Bateson, Don Jackson, Paul Watzlawick, John Weakland, Virginia Satir, Jay Haley and others. The Mental Research Institute proposed a model that 'normalised' and moved away from the 'illness' based view of mental health problems (Watzlawick, Weakland & Fisch, 1974).

Other therapies such as narrative and solution focus (Eron & Lund, 1996; Madigan & Epston, 1995; Walters & Peller, 2000) were gaining in popularity. The focus was beginning to shift towards what people did to maintain problem states and towards their strengths and abilities rather than their deficits and weaknesses.

▶ Brief therapy

These approaches have gradually percolated into the UK and Europe. They build on the main idea that the client has the resources needed to change and therapy focuses on accessing the strengths and abilities of the clients rather than focusing on what the client perceives as the problem. The attention is directed onto the desired outcome and various approaches are used to help the client begin to move towards their desired goal.

Brief therapy contrasted greatly with the psychoanalytic approaches prevalent at the time of its inception. Therapy had been viewed as always lengthy, sometimes lifelong, and most approaches did indeed seem to take a long time to achieve successful outcomes. People worked under the precept that change takes a long time to occur and so it did. Remember the four-minute mile? It was thought, and scientists proved, that it was physically and physiologically impossible for the human body to run a mile in under four minutes, but once Roger Bannister had done so, many people quickly followed suit. If you know how, there are many ways to help people change that do not need to take a huge amount of time from the busy health professional. After all, how fast is thought? The mind only works quickly.

As Milton Erickson believed 'What is needed is the development of a therapeutic situation permitting the client to use his own thinking, his own understandings, his own emotions in a way that fits him in his scheme of life' (Erickson, 1980).

Many therapists and scholars have studied Milton Erickson's work to try and discover the 'key' to his success as a therapist. Steve de Shazer described how he sorted Erickson's cases into six piles based on similar patterns or approaches ... but whatever parameters he used, the sixth pile was always the largest, and that was labelled 'miscellaneous', where each case intervention was unique (Shazer, 1994).

▶ The solution-focused approach

The solution-focused approach is utilisation: exploring a client's resources, experiences and skills ... 'then utilising these uniquely personal internal resources to achieve therapeutic goals' (Erickson & Rossi, 1979). This is also true of the human givens approach (for more information see www.humangivens.com) whereby people are seen to have innate resources to obtain various inbuilt needs and emotional distress occurs when these needs are not fulfilled.

Solution-focused, brief therapy (SFBT), NLP, hypnotherapeutic and the human givens approaches evolved within a clinical context and there are many anecdotal reports of success from both therapists and clients, but there is little in the way of controlled empirical evidence. Often these approaches seem to reduce the time needed to obtain a successful outcome and so are ideally suited to becoming incorporated into primary care where time is at a premium.

In 2000, Gingerich and Eisengart published a systematic review of 15 controlled outcome studies of SFBT. Five studies were well-controlled and all showed positive outcomes – four found SFBT to be better than no treatment or standard institutional services, and one found SFBT to be comparable to a known intervention: interpersonal psychotherapy for depression (IPT). Findings from the remaining 10 studies, which were considered moderately or poorly controlled, were consistent with a hypothesis of SFBT effectiveness.

There has been much evidence that hypnotic approaches are helpful in the management of many conditions ranging from dermatological, psychosomatic and psychological to acute and chronic pain. (Flammer & Bongartz, 2003; Montgomery et al., 2002). There is much in the literature to support the use of hypnotic approaches in pain (Montgomery, Duhamel & Redd, 2000; Sellick & Zaza, 1998; Syrjala, Cummings & Donaldson, 1992) to mention but a few and meta-analysis has demonstrated its effectiveness in therapy when combined with cognitive–behavioural approaches (Kirsch, Montgomery & Sapirstein, 1995). A general text such as Hartland's Medical and Dental Hypnosis 4th Edition gives numerous references for those interested but much of the evidence is based on cohort or case studies rather than random controlled trials (RCTs).

Personally, I find that William O'Hanlon's solution-oriented hypnosis approach melds brief solution focus work with hypnosis in a very effective way (O'Hanlon & Martin, 1992).

▶ On evidence

The gold standard for evidence-based medicine is based on evaluation by Random Controlled Trials (RCTs). These are the epitome of good scientific research, developed in medicine to evaluate physical treatments and then used by psychiatry to evaluate efficacy of medication. So the methodology used in drug research is applied to evaluate psychotherapy.

RCTs, by their very nature, have to have a vigorously controlled and regulated environment, type of client, amount of treatment and standardised interventions. They compare effect of an active drug with an inert placebo for a specific illness. Reduction of symptoms beyond that found with the placebo defines the efficacy of the drug.

Standardisation of therapy gives poorer results and undermines the therapeutic alliance (Castonguay *et al.*, 1996) and it has been shown that using psychodynamic therapy following a manual gave poorer results (Henry *et al.*, 1993) than when practised without.

So in many ways RCTs are inadequate for empirically validating psychotherapy as practised in reality (Seligman, 1995). How can we assess psychological interventions in such a way when therapy is not of fixed duration and clients often have multiple problems? Also therapy is far from standardised, therapists changing unsuccessful techniques and replacing them with others, according to the response of their client.

Clients often actively choose their therapist and therapeutic model and this has important implications as regards motivation and trust. Trials involving therapy needs huge numbers to obtain statistical significance with the number of variables involved (in drug trials psychological factors are dismissed as 'noise').

There is also the difficulty (ethically and otherwise) of having a placebo group. Clients may drop out and be a confounding variable and just being assigned in a trial may have an effect on the client and skew results. As mentioned in Chapter 1, the placebo effect is very important and may well account for a large percentage of successful outcome.

Therapist variables also need to be addressed. Clients may be randomised – but what about the therapists? Rosenthal and Rubin (1978) found that the 'Investigators' theoretical positions, beliefs and "expectancy effects" could even influence the behaviour of albino rats as well as children in controlled laboratory experiments with randomly selected subjects'.

Glenys Parry, Professor in Applied Psychological Therapies at Sheffield University, has stated 'Most psychological therapy in the NHS is pragmatic and eclectic. If delivered by skilled therapists this is based on sound psychological principles and flexibly tailored to the individual's needs. . . . By their very nature, randomised trials deprive clients of choice . . . research evidence of efficacy does not guarantee delivery of clinically effective therapies'.

It has been said that 'Guidelines are tools designed for the high ground of technical rationality, not the swamp where most primary care occurs' (Schon, 1983). Guidelines have their place in encouraging safe and ethical practice but slavish adherence to protocols and guidelines saps enthusiasm and creativity and ultimately does not benefit either health professional or client.

So how can we know what approaches or models 'work'?

▶ Practice-based evidence

Clients are in a context. We need to shift emphasis from does it work, to under what circumstances does it work, with whom, where, and when. Within the field of therapy and psychology, I believe we need practice-based evidence rather than evidence-based practice. We need to do outcome audit whenever possible.

An observation of a behaviour, e.g. someone shouting to another, may be quantified but can be given a very different qualitative assessment. The feelings will be very different if the shouting is set within a context of conflict or if the person shouting is trying to warn someone of danger.

So, given that we need to tailor our approach to the client, we also need to measure progress and outcomes in some way – to know that we are being effective in the work that we do. If we are not being effective – we need to know and then explore the reasons why. Too many people engage with therapy or counselling where no outcome measures are ever recorded.

The Clinical Outcomes for Routine Evaluation (CORE) is a useful outcome assessment tool that comprises 32 questions designed by the Psychological Therapies Research Centre, Leeds University in 1999 to evaluate client's feelings of well-being, perception of problems, how well they are functioning and risk of self-harm or harm to others. This is combined with various other forms and widely used within the UK (Evans *et al.*, 2000; Mellor-Clark *et al.*, 1999).

However, the supplementary forms are very subjective, based mainly on the therapist's opinions, and I feel are not particularly helpful, so a colleague of mine, Dr Ibbotson, devised an Excel spreadsheet, which is quickly completed and displays a graph of initial and final CORE scores. This gives an easy visual representation of how a client is progressing and as the CORE questionnaire is in the public domain, both this and the Excel spreadsheet is available to any therapist from our websites (geoff@geoffibbotson.co.uk or www.annwilliamson.co.uk).

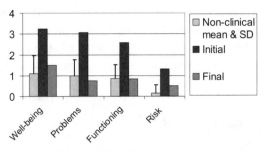

Figure 2.3 Example of a CORE graph

Client assessment is probably more valid than that of the therapist. Data from 40 years of outcome research show that it is the client, not the therapist that makes treatment work (Hubble, Duncan & Miller, 1999; Orlinsky, Grawe & Park, 1994).

Many health professionals in primary care use a shorter questionnaire – the Hospital Anxiety and Depression Scale (HADS) but this has to be purchased – it is not in the public domain. Other assessment tools such as the General Health Questionnaire (GHQ) are also commonly used.

Some form of analogue scale can be used to assess a client's emotional well-being and functioning such as the scaling question (see page ••) or the control centre imagery described in Chapter 11. Analogue scales of various kinds can also be used to assess satisfaction with the consultation or period of therapy.

Using some kind of measurement, whether it be quantitative or qualitative, is extremely important, otherwise we may find ourselves having spent all our time climbing a ladder – only to find that it is leaning on the wrong wall . . .

▶ Moving the client from problem to solution

'As long as therapeutic encounters focus on client's experiences as evidence of illness or pathology, then they remain trapped in pathology frames' where they 'are able to make sense of their experiences within that framework' (Asen *et al.*, 2004, p. 40).

Clients are experts on their problems and if they continually focus on the problem without thinking about solutions, then it can be useful to interrupt the pattern. This interruption of problem-based talk needs to be done in such a way so as not to break rapport. One way is by dropping a pen and bending down to pick it up or having a coughing fit. Then you need to come in with a solution-oriented comment or question to begin to turn the tide within the next second or two.

> ### Coughing fit – then
>
> 'Sorry about that – now I notice that you mentioned that you felt better last week – have you any ideas about how you did that?'

Turning towards a solution focus can begin with the first question in a consultation. 'What has already started to change since you made the decision to make this appointment?' Very often, things have started to move while the client has been waiting to see you.

> 'What has already started to change since you made the decision to make this appointment?'

Rather than 'What can I do for you today?', how about 'So what are we going to look at doing today that might be helpful?', which puts a collaborative slant on the consultation rather than the health professional being 'the expert' with all the answers.

▶ Balancing validation with a solution focus

Therapeutic history taking involves validating the client's distress but balancing that with the start of a shift towards solutions. If the health professional, while listening to the history, marks a client's strengths, and the times when the client has done something helpful, with tonality or remarks, it reinforces the shift from problem to solution focus. Asking the right kind of questions can help the consultation move towards solution orientation. Asking about achievements, enquiring about exceptions to the problem and finding out what has worked as solution in the past are all questions that move the history taking from mere fact finding to being therapeutic in its own right.

Elicit and Mark the Client's Strengths

What have they achieved in the past?

When does the problem NOT occur?

When is the problem less?

What has been used as solutions to similar problems in the past?

▶ **Summary**

Outcome audit improves practice and helps monitor progress with the client.

1. CORE

2. HADS

3. GHQ

4. Analogue scales

Therapeutic history taking

1. Take an initial record of emotional distress, e.g. with CORE or analogue scale

2. Balance validation of distress with solution focus

3. Build rapport

4. Interrupt prolonged problem focused talk

5. Elicit goals

6. Contract length and frequency of contact

7. Elicit client's strengths

CHAPTER THREE

How do we 'think'?

▶ Imagery

Imagery and metaphor are integral to how we think and how we construct and communicate our reality. When one starts to look at thought and how we construct our inner reality one has to consider imagery (Thomas, 2005). Jung says that the 'emotionally infused image is the primary organiser of the human psyche' (Young-Eisendrath & Hall, 1991). Freud (1923/1960) thought that thinking in pictures reflected unconscious processing more nearly than thinking in words.

How do we know that what we call a 'chair' is a 'chair'? We take what we see and compare it internally to other objects that we have labelled as 'chair'. At some level, we have an 'image' of a 'chair'. But the images we produce are very individual. We may be in basic agreement as to what constitutes a 'chair' but the images may range from a wooden kitchen chair, to an armchair to a wheelchair, depending on the context and the experiences of the person. This has relevance to our communications with our clients in that we need to be sure that the words we use evoke the same images in our clients as ourselves and that we are aware of what our client means by certain words or phrases.

Words that do not paint a picture in our minds invoke little emotion. The word 'sunset' of itself means nothing, unless I relate it internally to an image of the sunset with the colours streaking the sky. We will talk more on this later when we come to look at anchors in Chapter 12.

Jung maintained that thinking in images from a developmental viewpoint is prior to the mastery of language and syntax. He also felt that images are more powerful and motivating than language and that we use images to convey meaning and emotion that extends beyond that which can be encompassed by mere words. 'Metaphor flows from affect (emotion) because it usually represents the need to articulate a pressing inner experience of oneself and of one's internalised objects. It typically arises when feelings are high and when ordinary words do not seem strong enough or precise enough to convey the experience' (Siegelman, 1990, p. 16).

Imagery is frequently thought of as visual, and although the visual component is often predominant, imagery may also be auditory, olfactory/gustatory and kinaesthetic and I would also include spatial. Sometimes clients have an 'awareness' of whatever they are thinking about and know where in space it seems to be without actually having a visual image. When using imagery in therapy, all forms of processing need to be utilised.

▶ Models

A model is a representation of a process, often using metaphor, in order to improve understanding. It is virtually impossible to communicate concepts without the use of models or metaphor. However, difficulties start to arise if we start to believe our models are the 'Truth'.

Right/left brain model

One of the models commonly used to help explain why we often cannot change a negative emotional state simply by knowing 'intellectually' what to do or not to do is that of right and left-brain functioning, which can be seen as analogous to the conscious/unconscious model of mind.

Jerre Levy and Sperry showed that the right-brain processing is rapid, complex, whole-pattern, spatial and perceptual, whereas the left-brain processing is verbal and analytical. She (JL) found evidence that there was interference between these differing processing modes and then postulated that this may be a rationale for the evolutionary development of asymmetry in the human brain – as a means of keeping the two different modes of processing in two different hemispheres (Levi-Agreasti, 1968)

A useful, albeit rather basic, view of the differences in functioning can be seen below (Edwards, 1993).

Left hemispherical mode of functioning	Right hemispherical mode of functioning
Verbal – uses words to name and describe.	**Non-verbal** – awareness of things – *minimal connection with words*
Analytic – figures things out step by step	**Synthetic** – puts things together to form wholes
Symbolic – uses a symbol to stand for something	**Concrete** – relates to things as they are at the present moment
Abstract – takes a small bit of information and uses it to represent the whole	**Analogic** – sees likenesses between things, understands metaphorical relationships
Temporal – keeps track of time, sequences one thing after another	**Non-temporal** – without a sense of time
Rational – draws conclusions based on reasons and fact	**Non-rational** – not requiring a basis of fact – willingness to suspend judgement
Digital – uses numbers as in counting	**Spatial** – sees where things are in relation to each other, how things fit to form a whole
Logical – draws conclusions using sequential logic	**Intuitive** – makes leaps of insight, often on incomplete patterns, feelings or images
Linear – thinks in terms of linked ideas	**Holistic** – Sees whole things all at once perceiving overall patterns and structures

Left-brain functioning can be seen as analogous to our conscious awareness and right-brain functioning to our unconscious processing. As with all models, there are only some elements of 'truth' in this but it is a useful simplification.

Word pictures can be thought of as integrating non-linear/imaginal components with linear/verbal communication or, using the right and left brain model, they can be seen as communicating to both right and left brain, to both conscious and unconscious. For more on this model see Chapter 10.

▶ Metaphor

Since the 1970s, it became recognised that metaphors are a pervasive form of language, not just found in poetry and that they are in fact the root of creativity and an essential aspect of cognition (Winner, 1988).

Metaphoric communication has the ability to contemplate similarities and make a picture that conveys the meaning (Ricoeur, 1979). It is mostly non-literal and often used when you can't find the right word to describe something (Langer, 1942/1979).

Content (imagery) of metaphor is processed within the right hemisphere whereas the structure and form contained in the words is processed in the left hemisphere (Danesi, 1989). Therefore, metaphors need the functioning of both right and left hemispheres to be decoded both abstractly and conceptually so that their meaning can be understood. It acts as a link between left and right hemispheres, between intellectual rationality and emotional knowing.

When we think of any great teacher we find that they use metaphor and parable. They tell a story that invokes images within the listener. They take something that is unknown and graft it creatively onto something familiar.

Telling a story is a more powerful and a more memorable way of communicating than a simple statement of fact. In a therapeutic context, patterns of behaviour and relationships often need a language other than logic.

Myths and legends have been used from earliest times to communicate and preserve important information.

'Traditional knowledge handed down from generation to generation helped to save ancient tribes on India's Andaman and Nicobar Islands from the worst of the tsunami, anthropologists say'. In the path of the Tsunami in 2004, there were few fatalities because their myths and stories told them that when the gods drew back the sea it meant they had to flee into the mountains. When they saw the waters retreat from their shores, they heeded the story and ran inland away from the oncoming wave and were saved (Subir Bhaumik – BBC News online 20 January 2005).

Research on imaginal cognition and reflections of creative physicists support the view that imaginal cognition is essential to the creation of new ways of looking at things (Miller, 1986) so 'metaphoric interventions are especially well suited to the therapeutic task of creating new patterns and connections' (Kopp, 1995).

Client-generated metaphor

We all use metaphor to try and explain things, to convey meaning and emotion.

> 'He's like a bear with a sore head!'.
> 'She's like a bull in a china shop'.
> 'He really gets under my skin'.

These are all analogies; one of the simplest types of metaphorical statement, when we compare one thing to another.

Language reflects our internal reality and therefore is probably the most important tool we have to help people change.

The metaphors our clients use can often give us, as therapists, a powerful way of communicating with our client and helping them to access the changes that they desire.

This can be how the client views a problem: for instance, 'a can of worms', 'a pain in the neck', 'I feel trapped'. They can also be generated by such questions as: 'If I were seeing it (the problem) what would I see?'

These metaphors can be explored to good effect with further (non-leading) questions: 'What do you see as you experience that pain in the neck? What else do you see, what else is going on?' Other senses may then be introduced: 'What does it sound/feel like to be 'trapped'?' and then a beneficial change is suggested: 'If you could make one change to it in some way, what would you do?' We will expand on these approaches in subsequent chapters.

Case 1: David

> 'It's as though I know what I need to do but there's a brick wall in the way'.

The session was spent exploring how he could get around, climb over or in some way get through to the resources he saw as available to himself on the other side of the wall. He finally decided that he would make the wall into an archway.

In this process, he was gaining acceptance of the obstacles in his path (the wall) rather than ignoring them (climbing over them) and was using his creativity to utilise the obstacles as a way to progress (making the bricks into an archway).

Using metaphors like this is one way of externalising the 'problem' so that rather being part of a person's identity, it becomes something that can be talked about and altered. It gives the client a different perspective on their problem and is extended further in gestalt and narrative therapy approaches.

Using imagery moves us from a logical–cognitive perspective to sensory–imaginal processing; from disembodied analytic thought processing to sensory–affective imagery and somatic experience.

▶ Memory

We store memories in different ways: a personal memory may be an image (of myself as a teenager walking over the rocks around a point with the wind and the sea spray in my face), an autobiographical event without an image, (when I received my medical degree), or more generic in type (walking through dry autumn leaves), which involves sensory information but not a specific time or event.

Memory is not reproductive – we do not have a video camera that records everything and replays it at will. Every time we remember something, we reconstruct the memory from various different bits of information that have been stored. Some pieces may be missing but our mind substitutes an approximation and this then becomes our 'memory'. From a therapeutic viewpoint, it does not matter whether the 'memory' that the client has is historically accurate – it is how their mind has constructed the problem and has to be worked with at that level. If one is working with past trauma, this is important as 'false memories' can easily be created by any leading questions or simply by implication. It is important that the client understands that what is being worked with as a 'past memory' may be a symbolic or metaphorical representation of the problem rather than historical 'fact'.

Empathic metaphor

Often when in good rapport with a client, the therapist may find a story, metaphor or idea popping into their mind as the client talks and this can also be utilised. 'May I tell you the image that occurred to me when you were saying . . .?' You can then check whether the images conjured up in your mind are relevant to the client and help them to see the problem differently.

Constructed metaphor

Stories, fairy tales, myths and legends can act as a bridge to help us access a child's ability to learn; they can remind us of possibilities and options and show us different perceptions. The aim of any therapeutic intervention is to connect the client with a different, more helpful perspective than they originally had and imagery and metaphor can be a powerful way of doing this in an unthreatening but highly effective manner.

Any good storyteller knows that it is the descriptive words that give a story its power to connect with the listener's imagination. One paints a picture in words but also utilises the other senses such as sound, smell and touch.

Clients typically make a link between their past sensory and perceptual experience and metaphoric statements (Verbrugge & McCarrel, 1977). They interpret the metaphor in their own individual way and take the meaning that is relevant to them.

Another possible reason for the power of metaphorical communication is that it can bypass a client's conscious resistance or defenses to change and allow the suggestion of change to be accepted as it is presented in a non-threatening way.

Constructed metaphor combines layers of meaning, inherent in the words and metaphors used, with a story that allows the message to be a communication to the client at an unconscious level. The therapeutic power is increased by allowing less precision in assigning meaning to the story by the therapist, allowing the client to choose the most useful interpretation for themselves (Kopp, 1995).

Constructed metaphors may be stories from the therapists own background and experience. They may also be about nature or types of experience that are so universal that the client cannot deny them or more complicated stories designed to make a point. These may be metaphors that the therapist has constructed previously, designed and tailor-made for a particular client; or ones that are in the therapist's repertoire that are applicable to certain situations or types of problem.

Experiential metaphor

One can use simple everyday objects to make a point to your clients experientially. We will give many examples of these in succeeding chapters. All the creative arts can be used as forms of experiential metaphor. Dance movement, music and art are all used in therapy to explore a difficulty metaphorically and then to connect the client with their inner ways of helping, their strengths or their desired state.

▶ Association and dissociation

It is important to understand the difference between an associated and a dissociated image. In an associated image, it is as if you were actually there and reliving the experience. If you are having an associated recollection of a ride on a roller coaster, you can see the view from the roller coaster, hear the sounds, feel the wind and feel the movement in your body. Association makes the experience real and amplifies the effect of the event. The more of the sensory systems that are activated the more realistic the experience.

A dissociated image would involve you seeing yourself on the roller coaster – as though on a video but with none of the experiential information or emotional impact from being on the ride.

Because associated imagery increases the effect, it is used in this way when you want to help a client connect with positive feelings. Dissociated imagery decreases affect and so can be used in this way when working with negative and traumatic memories.

While taking a history, one should encourage associated recollections of positive experiences and avoid associating the client into negative experiences.

If a client is becoming associated into a negative experience, then techniques, such as pattern interrupts, are very useful in order to break into the associated negative experience as mentioned already in Chapter 2. In these circumstances, it is possible to drop a pen, or suddenly remember that a questionnaire 'has' to be completed, in order to act as an informal 'pattern interrupt' or 'break state'.

A Caveat

Unless you are trained and used to working with psychotic clients, you should not attempt imagery and visualisation work with anyone who is actively psychotic as they already have difficulty separating reality from fantasy.

▶ **Summary**

- Imagery can be:

  1. visual

  2. auditory

  3. kinaesthetic

  4. olfactory

  5. gustatory

  6. spatial

- Word pictures, such as those generated in stories and metaphors, integrate right and left brain modes of processing, conscious and unconscious, linear verbal and non-linear sensory, imaginal forms of processing. This helps to link intellectual rationality with emotional knowledge and understanding.

- Memory is seldom historically accurate but needs to be worked with as a representation of what a certain event 'meant' to the client.

- Metaphors can be:

  1. empathic

  2. constructed

  3. experiential

- Association with an image or memory means the client is, in effect, reliving and re-experiencing the event, which increases the affect. This should be encouraged when getting the client to access a positive feeling.

- Dissociation from an image or memory means that the client is watching themselves 'from outside' and this decreases affect. This should be encouraged when the client is accessing a traumatic memory.

- Do not use imagery with clients who have an active psychosis.

CHAPTER FOUR

Building rapport

▶ What do we mean by rapport?

How many of us enjoy being told what to do? If we are told that some habit or behaviour we have is bad for us and that we should change it how do we respond? Many people start to justify their behaviour, which only serves to re-enforce it, and no one changes unless they feel that they wish to do so for their own reasons.

If you do not build rapport but simply tell the client something, whether trying to help them with an emotional state, or give them lifestyle advice, you might as well save your breath and not bother! Unless suggestions are given in rapport, they are unlikely to be effective in helping your client make the changes they want.

> You know smoking is very bad for you
> - Have you ever thought of stopping smoking?
> - You have got to stop!
> Which approach would you be more likely to respond to?

Occasionally, the direct command will work but more often it will be ignored. The more indirect approach within rapport is likely to be much more productive.

So what is rapport? At its most basic level, it means being interested in your client as a fellow human being. It means listening with 'a kindly eye and an open heart' and not having preconceived ideas and judgements about the client and their problems.

The Oxford dictionary definition of rapport mentions 'Sympathy; connection; an emotional bond'. That rapport is important when giving suggestion was recognised as early as 1948 when a dictionary definition said it was 'A state in which mesmeric action can be exer-

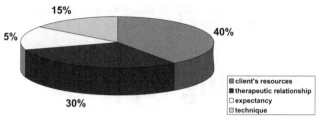

15%

5%

40%

30%

- client's resources
- therapeutic relationship
- expectancy
- technique

Figure 4.1 Influencing factors in change

cised by one person on another'. We may not all use formal hypnotic (mesmeric) techniques but we all, as health professionals, need to know how to give suggestion powerfully if we are to help people to have a healthier lifestyle or comply with treatment.

It has been shown that people with anxiety and depression benefit from psychotherapy (Strupp, 1996) and most studies find the average treated person is better off than 80% of those without treatment (Assay & Lambert, 1999).

There seem to be four categories of factors that influence change and contribute to positive outcome: client factors (resources) 40%; therapeutic relationship factors 30%; hope and expectancy 15% and model/technique 15% (Assay & Lambert, 1999; Lambert, 1992).

So it can be said that gaining good rapport with your client can be responsible for a third of the improvement seen. The therapist alliance and the quality of the therapeutic relationship is hugely important (Blatt *et al.*, 1996; Orlinsky, Grawe & Park, 1994).

By the therapeutic relationship I mean the relationship between client and health professional that is built up by listening, validating and encouraging the client to achieve their goals.

To a great extent, it doesn't matter what therapeutic approach or model is used (Wampold *et al.*, 1997). They all work because the client utilises what each approach offers to address their problems (Tallman & Bohart, 1999). If we focus on the client's strengths and resources within a consultation where we have good rapport and expect a positive outcome then we are 85% there.

Self-help may also be as effective as therapy – a study of a class of people with depression taught cognitive self-help procedures improved as much as those treated in a National Institute of Mental Health collaborative study in the States (Arkowitz, 1997).

▶ Pacing and leading

One way of looking at rapport is to see it as pacing and leading. You walk alongside the client (metaphorically speaking), pacing together, and then you can begin to lead. Often this process begins to happen naturally within a consultation but sometimes it helps to know ways to build rapport so that you can help the process along. The client also needs to determine the direction in which you both walk (see Chapter 5).

There are many ways that you can begin to pace your client but it has to be done with sensitivity or it can have the opposite effect.

Emotional pacing

The first step is to acknowledge and let the client know that you understand a little of how they are feeling – you can never know completely, as we are each unique human beings with different backgrounds, influences and internal processing, but we do have our own experiences to draw upon and we can all use our imagination to get some understanding of the client's difficulties.

You do not want to join them in their negative feelings but the client needs to feel that their feelings are valid. Tonality can be useful here – a strategically placed 'Hm', or 'Yes, I can see that', or maybe reflecting back to the client their words or phrases.

Posture pacing

It can be helpful to match or mirror your client's posture. Often an anxious client will be sitting tensely on the edge of their chair and you can match this by sitting upright and then as you begin to sit back more comfortably, the client will follow suit if you are in rapport.

If they move then you can move in a similar manner within a few seconds. For instance, if they touch their ear, then you could touch your throat or neck chain. The client will notice at an unconscious level and feel that you are 'with them'. This happens quite spontaneously as you can see if you 'people watch' in a restaurant or bar. But one does need to be a little subtle about this. If you copied slavishly every move your client made, then this could have the opposite effect as it would be noticed consciously and probably misinterpreted as mockery.

Pacing breathing

One of the most powerful ways to build rapport is by matching the client's breathing rate. If the client's breathing is very fast, this could be uncomfortable, so a way around this is to make some other movement (e.g. tapping finger) at the same rate. This is called crossmatching. Once one has built rapport you can begin to lead, maybe slowing down your breathing rate gradually as the client follows suit.

Pacing language

One can also begin to notice the language the client is using, reflecting back words or phrases as appropriate. Notice and use the client's language. We all use all our senses at various times and when we speak we often use language that reflects our favourite method of sensing at the time. This is called our representational system. Our main representational systems are auditory, visual and kinaesthetic and these are reflected in our language.

Words people use can be auditory in style 'I hear what you are saying', 'It sounds very difficult'. They could be visual 'I see what you mean', 'It seems to me', 'The future looks black' or kinaesthetic 'It's weighing me down', 'I feel so wound up'.

It has been shown that positive client satisfaction is related to the therapist having a similar linguistic style to the client (Patton & Meara, 1982). If you respond to 'I keep getting a sinking feeling whenever I think about it' (kinaesthetic) with 'I think you need to look at all the alternatives' (visual), it is as though you are responding in French to Spanish! You can build rapport by using a similar sense style in your language to the client. This may seem difficult at first but with a little practice it soon becomes easier.

Voice pacing

Matching tone and tempo of someone's speech can also help build rapport but beware of seeming to appear mocking. When I speak to someone with a Celtic accent, I automatically tend to lapse into the accent and have had to apologise in advance on several occasions in case I gave offence!

This may all seem very contrived and complicated but understanding a little of how people build rapport between each other can be useful if you are working with someone that you don't immediately 'take to'.

By pacing and building rapport over the first few minutes of a consultation – maybe by matching body language and acknowledging the client's emotional state – you build an environment in which the client, at an unconscious level, feels safe and valued and which is far more likely to lead to useful communication.

Begin to notice the language your client uses – it can tell you much more than the sense of the words they are using. Often clients will tell you quite unconsciously how to help them.

Types of Pacing

1. Emotional . . . acknowledge

2. Posture . . . mirror/match

3. Breathing . . . pace rate/cross-match

4. Language . . . representational systems; mainly auditory, kinaesthetic, visual

5. Voice . . . tone/tempo

Eye-accessing cues

I will also, for completeness, mention here eye-accessing cues. These have been extensively studied in NLP but I think are of little relevance to the practising health professional except in a very limited way. As a general rule, people's eyes flick upwards if they are seeing something 'in their mind's eye', to the side if they are imagining hearing something and downwards if they are feeling something or talking to themselves (internal dialogue). If you notice this, it can sometimes

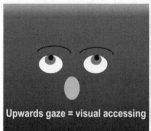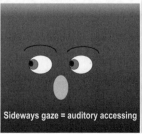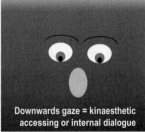

Upwards gaze = visual accessing | Sideways gaze = auditory accessing | Downwards gaze = kinaesthetic accessing or internal dialogue

Figure 4.2 Eye-accessing cues

give you insight into how the client is constructing their reality at the time. For instance, if you ask a question and you notice the client's eyes flick up as they consider their answer you could ask 'How does that look?'. This would of course help build rapport as you are acknowledging the client's processing.

Body language

Watch your client's body language; a change as they are talking may be very significant and point out something that is important or that they are having difficulty with. Up to 70% of our communication takes place at the non-verbal level so body language is extremely important and is not easily faked. The non-verbal will often come prior to the verbal response and minimal changes in facial muscle tone can alert you to the important parts of whatever someone is telling you. Asymmetry in body posture can alert you to possible conflicts within the individual as can incongruity between the verbal communication and the accompanying body language. Non-verbal feedback whilst taking a history from a client can alert you and indicate a sensitive area. The decision whether to explore this or not would depend on time and the degree of rapport between client and health professional. Sometimes it may be necessary to take a note and explore it at a subsequent appointment.

Normalising and validating a person's experience and letting the client know that you accept them, that 'I'm on your side, I believe in you' is paramount in any effective consultation.

> The most important way of building rapport is to be genuinely interested in the client you are with at the time and to allow them to express how they feel, think and behave in a non-judgemental atmosphere of caring.

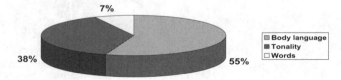

7%

38%   55%

■ Body language
■ Tonality
□ Words

Figure 4.3 Communication (Mehrabian, 1971)

▶ Summary

Rapport = pacing . . . and then leading.

Types of pacing:

1. Posture

2. Movement

3. Breathing

4. Voice

5. Language

Representational systems:

1. Visual . . . I see what you mean

2. Auditory . . . That sounds good to me

3. Kinaesthetic . . . I have a gut feeling

Exercise

Next time a very anxious client comes into your consulting room why not notice their body language and gradually pace them for a while. When you feel that you have got rapport, test it and see if as you relax your posture a little, they follow your lead.

CHAPTER FIVE

Goal setting

▶ Expectancy

As has been mentioned earlier, expectancy effects are important for positive outcomes. If a client does not believe that change is possible then they are probably correct, although sometimes the health professional needs to 'carry hope for people when they can't carry it for themselves' (Rapp & Goscha, 2006).

If you, the health professional, believe that your client has abilities and resources that will enable them to make the changes that they wish, then your focus will be in enhancing such skills and kindling in your client an expectation that they can succeed. This works 'with the person's natural energy for recovery, rather than wasting energy on trying to convince (or at worst coerce) a person to do something the client does not want, which often leads to undue resistance, tension within the helping relationship, or passive acceptance' (Rapp & Goscha, 2006, p. 62).

Hope is the key to a successful outcome. If a person has no hope then the chances are that they will give up and do nothing because what is the point if nothing is going to work?

We invest more energy in doing things we enjoy or do well and often tend to avoid things we do, or think we do, badly. Finding out what your client does well means that you can reflect back to them their strengths.

Case 2: Maureen

Maureen suffered with chronic recurrent depression and low levels of confidence and self-esteem. I discovered that she was very keen on doing cross stitch. She brought in a sample of her work, an elaborate and painstakingly made picture of a rural farm scene. As we looked at it together I asked her to tell me what skills she needed to accomplish this work. Among others we listed persistence, ability to concentrate, attention to detail, dexterity, an eye for colour and a love of beautiful things. This acknowledgement (by her) of some of her strengths was one of her first steps to believing in herself.

Find ways of generating hope and expectancy in your client. This may be by seeding ideas (see Chapter 8), by talking about your own experiences or by talking about some other client with a similar difficulty and how they managed to achieve their goals.

Another way of generating expectancy can be by getting the client to realise that they have not always had these problems and to look at times when either the problem didn't arise, didn't arise when expected or had less of an impact (see pages 28 & 66). What was happening then that was different?

▶ Defining a goal

Clients are experts at their problems but may find it difficult to envisage solutions. Often they can be very vague about what they want to do or feel. As health professionals, it is part of our job to help clients determine their goals. Goals need to be specific. I usually ask my clients to imagine seeing themselves on a video and tell me what they are doing once their problem has resolved and they are feeling the way they want to be.

How will you know when you've got there?
How will others know when you've got there?

Another way of achieving this is by asking the client to use their imagination and engage their unconscious resources by closing their eyes and visualising the future the way they would like it to be. One way of eliciting goals can be with the 'Miracle Question' and clients often find it easier to generate an answer if they close their eyes, relax and visualise themselves in an associated way (see page 38) actually getting up in the morning, etc.

The Miracle Question

I would like to ask you now to close your eyes and imagine that you are going to bed. You get in and snuggle down under the bedclothes feeling comfortable, warm and drowsy. (Give them a little time to engage with these suggestions.) Gradually, you fall asleep and while you are asleep, a miracle happens and your difficulties are resolved. But you are asleep and do not realise this. I would then like you to imagine waking up the next morning. When you wake up what is the first thing that would tell you that something had happened? What would you notice that would be different? How would those around you know something was different?

If a client really cannot formulate a goal then at the very least they must have a direction and one can work towards that, maybe formulating a goal later.

If you order a taxicab the first thing the driver asks is 'Where do you want to go?'

If a goal seems vague, the health professional needs to dig for further information. What does that vague goal actually mean to the client? What would they be doing/thinking/feeling? Have they ever felt like that in the past? What was happening then? Sometimes it can be helpful to ask if they know someone who has achieved the goal they want for themselves and if so to ask how they know that that person has achieved it.

> ### *A Vague Goal – 'I Want to Be Happy'*
>
> You need more specific information:
>
> 'What does being happy mean to you?'
> 'Have you ever felt like that? What was happening then?'
> 'Do you know someone who is happy? What makes you think they're happy?'

▶ Motivation

To be motivated to achieve a goal, the person needs to feel that the goal is possible, worthwhile and that it is something that they want for themselves. Goals set by others do not motivate. If a client is coming to see you because they think they 'ought to' or someone else has pushed them into coming to see you then take time to ensure that the goal you elicit is really something they want for themselves or you will waste your time and theirs. Some people actually do not want to move from where they are.

> **If you don't have a direction or a goal, do you really want to go anywhere?**

Goals are cognitive representations of a future event and, bearing in mind what has been said about the use of imagery, are far more powerful if visualised. Having a goal gives purpose, helps mobilise the client's strengths and abilities needed to achieve the goal and engenders motivation and drive. Engaging with a person's creativity means that obstacles are more easily overcome as their approach may be more flexible.

▶ Visualising goals

There are two caveats to getting clients to visualise the way they want to be. Sometimes people have difficulty in visualising themselves. If this is merely because they are not good at visual imagery it doesn't matter at all – suggest that they get an 'awareness' of how they want to be, not necessarily visually, when you say 'see' or 'imagine'.

The other difficulty may be that they have a problem in actually imagining being the way they want to be because it is so far away from where they feel right now. In this case, the scaling question can be very useful.

▶ **Scaling question**

Ask the client to imagine some kind of a line or scale with themselves the way they would like to be at 10 with the opposite at 0 and imagine where they are now on that continuum. People tend to have a very clear idea of where they are and it is surprisingly specific. Then ask them to see what they would need to do or think differently to move up by one step to their goal of 10. I encourage them to be very specific and write their answers down so that we can check how they have got on in the next week or two.

Case 2: Maureen

Maureen felt that she was at about 4 on her scale. She said that what was keeping her from a 3 was telephoning her friend and having a chat each day; she decided that going out for a short walk each day would move her up to a 5.

Suggesting that they close their eyes and 'go inside' to experience a response to the question may help as also does asking them to imagine a video of themselves getting up one morning at 5 on their scale and noticing what was different to how they did it today at 4. The other useful information they can get from this scaling question is to look at what they are doing now that is stopping them from sliding further down the scale to 3.

Some health professionals seem to feel that 'allowing' their client to set goals can be setting up the client to fail. If the health professional feels that certain goals seem unrealistic or could lead to worsen-

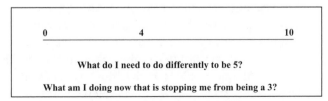

Figure 5.1 Example of the scaling questions with the client at '4'

ing of the client's problems, it is important not to rubbish them. More information is needed. What does that goal actually 'mean' to the client, what is its significance? Goals need to be accepted and explored – not debated.

▶ The 'experimental' approach

Trying things out 'as an experiment' means there is no pass or fail and this can often be a useful way of framing things (see Chapter 9).

> ### *Case 3: Amy*
>
> Amy, an intelligent 19-year-old, suffered with panic disorder and agarophobia but wanted to be able to go to college. She had not been out walking from her house for more than a year and thought she would feel too anxious.
>
> Having taught her some ways of coping with anxiety, we decided she would experiment and see how many lampposts she could walk from home. Once she started to feel anxious she would stop, calm herself and then retrace her steps. She surprised herself by finding that she could walk to the end of her road.

▶ Reinforcement

It is important that small successes are noted and commented upon as clients will often not notice that change is taking place. A sense of achievement follows such recognition which leads to increased motivation and confidence; a positive feedback loop.

> Sarah had long-standing depression and over the last six months had spent much of her time in bed trying to hide away from the world and herself. She rated herself at –1 on the scaling question until I pointed out to her that she had managed to get up, wash, get dressed, get in the car and come on time to her appointment. She acknowledged that this was an achievement and revised her score to 1. We then explored how she had managed to accomplish this.

Failure gives rise to feelings of powerlessness and frustration, which leads to decreased energy and motivation, and a lowering of confidence and hope; a negative feedback loop.

It is important therefore that goals are broken down into small achievable chunks and that 'failure' is reframed as a learning process.

Mistakes are an important way to learn.

Metaphor can be useful here and one I often use is that of learning to walk. This has a powerful message that behaviour takes time to change and that 'failure' should be regarded merely as a temporary setback.

▶ The walking/crawling metaphor
(This comes from Milton Erickson)

I ascertain whether the client used to crawl as a baby or shuffle along on their bottom and I then describe the process of learning to walk.

> When you were a toddler you probably crawled, that was how you got around. But then you started to pull yourself up onto your feet, swaying to get a feel for the right balance. After a while, when you had mastered that, you tried lifting one foot up and then putting it down a little further away. You then worked out how to take your weight on that leg while lifting the other and putting it down in front of you. You learnt to walk. But as you were learning, every now and then you lost your balance and fell down on your bottom and started to crawl again. Gradually, you crawled less and less and walked more and more, until now you only get down on all fours to crawl if you make a conscious decision to do so.

Successful goals require the client to be able to imagine them, to utilise the necessary skills and to have confidence that their goal is achievable.

Even small goals require effort and some people fail because they are feeling lazy and become easily discouraged. In this situation, the health professional needs to find out about times when goals were achieved in the past and what was different then.

▶ Learning skills

Sometimes there can be a mismatch between the goals people set themselves and their skills. But in this situation, we need to devise ways that the client can learn the skills that are needed. By engaging

GOAL SETTING

55

both the client's and the health professional's creativity, ways of doing this can usually be found.

> Twenty-two-year-old Pauline suffered with anxiety, panic attacks and agoraphobia. She wanted to work with children but realised that to do this she had to face her fears and go to college. She would also need to be able to cope with being interviewed. Among skills she identified as needing to achieve this was the ability to talk to someone without feeling anxious and panicky. Having worked successfully for some while on her panic attacks and agoraphobia, she decided to go and work in her brother's café waiting on tables so that she could get used to speaking to customers. She also practised going into shops and asking the shop assistants where various items were to be found until she felt comfortable doing this.

▶ Self-image

How we internally 'see' ourselves expresses itself in how we feel and behave.

An exercise that I often teach clients that is useful to improve their self-image or set a goal is the mirror exercise. If a client sees themselves in their mind's eye as stressed, anxious or depressed then they will tend to behave like that. If you can begin to focus them on how they want to be they will often start to begin to feel that way. It also helps to motivate a client towards a goal as they are visualising how they want to be.

> **You are whatever you think you are – if you change what you think, then you change what you are.**

▶ Mirror exercise

I ask them to close their eyes, settle down in whatever way they have found best and imagine behind themselves an image of how they don't want to be, a dull, unattractive image, feeling anxious, out of control and lacking in confidence. Then, in front, to imagine an image of themselves, looking, feeling, behaving, being the way they wish to be. I ask them choose which image they want to connect with. When they indicate the desired image in front I ask them to imagine stepping into the image in front, feeling it, noticing how good it feels and to say something appropriate to themselves, e.g. 'I'm glad I'm feeling calmer now' and then open their eyes. I ask them to repeat this four or five times, opening their eyes between each cycle until the image behind them fades or becomes less distinct. They could also do this with imagining themselves in some specific situation.

Effective suggestion needs the client to *associate* with their goal.

I usually suggest that the client do this exercise each morning upon waking so as to focus on where they want to go and to give themselves positive suggestion at the same time. This is especially useful when a client tells you that they 'Know what kind of a day I'm going to have as soon as I open my eyes!'

Brian was a 40-year-old dental phobic. Having done some work on his phobia, by the second session he was able to imagine himself sitting in the dental chair feeling reasonably calm and in control. I suggested that he do the mirror exercise daily – mirror behind with an image of Brian feeling anxious and panicky and a mirror in front with an image of him coping well with being in the dental chair – to 'step' into that image, feel how good it was to feel quite calm in that situation and to tell himself internally 'Wow! I can do this!' (he decided on the phrase he used). By then opening his eyes and repeating it 4–5 times, he was internally setting his goal, trying it out and connecting with his inner abilities to achieve this.

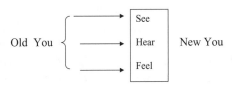

Figure 5.2   Minor exercise: associate with your goal

▶ The swish

A similar exercise known as the 'Swish' works in a similar way although here you imagine the undesirable 'Old you' on a screen in front of you with the 'New you' in a tiny image in the corner (rather like a computer icon). Expand the new image across the screen so that you can no longer see the old image and then push it back down into the icon. This is then repeated until it will no longer compress down and expose the old image. Once this stage has been reached it is a good idea to ask the client to imagine stepping into the new image, associate with it and experience it fully.

Alternatively, imagine the two images side by side and as you bring the 'New you' forward, push the 'Old you' image back into the distance.

All these techniques help to focus the client where they want to go and the more vividly they can imagine the 'New you' the stronger the positive suggestion they are giving themselves and the more they will get in touch with their unconscious resources. You see it, step into it and feel it, and say something positive about it to yourself, thus utilising all the senses.

▶ Smoking cessation

I often use this kind of technique to help smokers motivate themselves when they come to see me for help with smoking cessation. The 'Old you' behind coughing, spluttering and stinking like an old ashtray and the 'New you' in front, smelling fresh, feeling fitter and healthier and saying to someone 'I'm a non-smoker now' or 'I don't use those (cigarettes) anymore!'

▶ Positive mental rehearsal

It is also very useful for clients to use visualisation to 'try out' different goals. We all tend to set limits upon ourselves 'Oh! I can't do that!' but when we set a goal for ourselves using visualisation we do not have those conscious doubts to the same extent. If we can vividly imagine it and it feels right for us then all our unconscious resources and abilities will make it far more likely that we will achieve it.

▶ Ecology check

If they use some self-hypnotic technique and then vividly imagine the outcome they are exploring and step into it, they will get a sense of whether it is right for them as a whole person or not. It is important that the image in front feels right to the client, that it is ecological for them as a whole person within the context of their lives; if it is an unrealistic goal then they will not feel comfortable with it and will need to change it in some way. If it intuitively does not feel right then adjustments to the goal are needed until it does.

I usually suggest that clients do this exercise in their head but I find it is often more powerful to actually walk it out on the floor if the client is happy to do this. I find it is also a very useful way to help people get out of negative states if they feel 'stuck'.

▶ A goal-setting exercise

First, they stand up, this is position 1 – you, the way you are now ('Old you').

Now, in front of where they are standing, they imagine themselves the way they would like to be – this is position 2. Make it a really good feeling image ('New you').

Then they step to one side – position 3, where they can 'see' both images 1 and 2 ('Observer you'). From this position, they are in touch with all their unconscious resources. They can 'go inside' and as they look at '1' and '2', they can see exactly what they need in order to move from '1' to '2'. Allow their unconscious mind to gather up those resources and project them to 'Old you' in position 1.

They then move back to position 1 and accept the resources from their 'Observer' and integrate them fully into themselves.

Then they can move into position 2 feeling the way they want to feel, behaving the way they want to behave, and above all, feeling how good it is to be the way they want to be. They need to allow themselves a few moments to really experience this and then reorientate themselves back to the here and now, bringing with them all the good feelings they have just experienced.

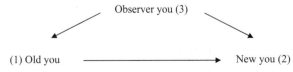

Figure 5.3 Perceptual positions

▶ Problem solving

Delving into why the client is suffering from anxiety or depression is of very limited value. Problem solving may be a first step but is certainly not the end of the journey.

It is the usual human approach that when we have a practical problem we analyse it, think about it and hopefully come up with solutions. Unfortunately, we often apply the same process to emotional problems, which, far from bringing solutions, tends to reinforce the problem and develop the negative emotional state further.

▶ New behaviours

Old patterns of behaviour may feel comfortable, like an old coat, but after a while you usually prefer to wear a new one! I also use the metaphor of buying a new pair of shoes. At first, they may feel a little strange and even a little uncomfortable but as you wear them they become a part of you and you don't even notice when you have them on your feet.

> **Goals need to be accepted and explored – not debated**
> **Why don't we try an experiment?**

▶ Summary

1. Generate expectancy.

2. Define a goal or at least a direction.

3. Associate the client in some way with the completed goal and check whether it is 'ecological' for them:

   ■ Miracle question

   ■ Scaling questions

   ■ Mirror exercise

   ■ Swish

   ■ Perceptual positions

4. Go for it!

Mirror exercise

1. Start with eyes closed
2. Image behind – the negative state
3. Image in front – the desired state
4. Step into the one you want – implication of choice but who wants the negative state?!
5. Feel how it feels to be 'x'
6. Say something appropriate to yourself
7. Open your eyes
8. Repeat 4–5 times

Principles of suggestion:

1. Repetition increases effectiveness
2. Vividness increases effectiveness
3. Strong emotion increases effectiveness
4. Positive phrasing increases effectiveness
5. If you think you can't – trying won't succeed!

◀ CHAPTER SIX ▶

Identity or behaviour?

When we feel depressed or anxious we often take on our emotional state as a way of being or identity. This is reflected in the language we use: 'I am depressed', 'I am anxious'. This is a very static state of affairs and leaves little room for change. If someone *is* depressed they feel as if they are stuck in that feeling forever.

▶ Thoughts, feelings and behaviour

One of the most important messages that we need to get across to our clients is that there is a continual cycle between our thoughts, behaviour and feelings. Emotional states don't just arise out of thin air – we create them by thinking and behaving in certain ways. If you can lead the client to realise that they are just *doing* depression for a while then this is a much more dynamic state of affairs. Emotions may be triggered by hot buttons but we can either fuel them, or not. Sights, smells, sounds can all trigger an emotional response (see Chapter 12 on anchoring) but we then develop and maintain the emotional state by how we then think and behave. There is a continual interplay and re-enforcement between our thoughts, behaviour and feelings.

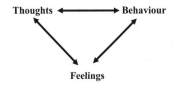

Figure 6.1   A continual feedback loop

Case 1: David

Upon asking David how he 'did' anxiety he determined that he first noticed a feeling or a twinge somewhere in his body. This led to catastrophising thoughts (see Chapter 7) such as 'I'm starting to be ill again!', 'I won't be able to . . .', 'Oh God, what's wrong?', which generated more feelings of fear and anxiety . . . and the pattern continued in an ever increasing negative spiral resulting in David withdrawing more and more and suffering increasing levels of anxiety and depression.

If they are *doing* something then there is always the possibility of doing it differently. It can give you a lever that you can use to help the client begin to feel differently.

▶ Eliciting change

The most important aim of brief psychological interventions is to lead the client to accept that there is **always change** and that they are visiting or doing, e.g. depression, anxiety, etc. for a time.

There are several ways in which we can begin to do this. While taking a history and talking to our client we can begin to change tense when reflecting back to the client – 'When you **were** depressed . . .' – 'You tell me that while you *have been* feeling anxious you were also having problems sleeping'.

They will not consciously notice the tense change but if accepted then the depression or the anxiety has been figuratively put into the past and they have accepted an unconscious suggestion that their emotional state is something that has not always been and will not always be . . . that it can change.

If you have good rapport you might try 'Well, I can see that you have been doing anxiety really well recently – lets begin to look at *how* you are doing it so well!'

If the health professional talks about 'the depression' or 'the anxiety', it starts to separate these emotional states from the client's sense of identity. As the emotional state is separated from the person, or externalised, it can be more easily discussed and it is easier for the client to gather different perspectives on the problem.

We can begin to mention limited periods of time when talking about how they feel 'When you were feeling depressed *last week* . . .'. We can begin to put some time limits on their distress.

This change in perception can also be helped by using experiential metaphors, an approach taught by the French Canadian therapist, Danie Beaulieu (2006):

> Susan had been feeling depressed and anxious for many months, in fact ever since her divorce two years before. She was a 37-year-old schoolteacher with a daughter aged nine. She came into the consulting room feeling despondent and hopeless. She tells me 'I don't seem able to pull myself out of feeling like this . . . every day is such a struggle . . . just to get through . . . there just seems no end to it'.
>
> I drew a line on a piece of paper representing her lifeline and asked Susan to mark when her depression had started to be a problem. She then realised that for the majority of her life to date she had not felt like this . . . she realised this far more powerfully seeing a visual representation than if we had just talked about it. This challenged her over generalisation and introduced time as an element of change.

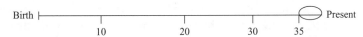

Birth |————————————————————————⊂⊃ Present
           10   20   30   35

Figure 6.2 Susan's lifeline.

Another way of achieving this change in perception is by using a piece of paper and marking it as in Figure 6.3 and then folding the paper so that the black part 'D' that represents the depression is folded back. As you turn the paper to present this black part to the client you ask 'Do you want to define yourself by this'; 'Do you only want to show the world only this part?'; and 'What about all the rest?' and turn the paper so that the white area shows.

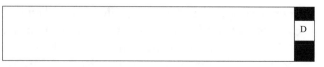

Figure 6.3 The black 'D' (depression) is a very small part of the whole.

▶ Exceptions

We can begin to find and mark exceptions – 'Were there days (or hours) when you felt calmer or less depressed?' . . . 'Have there been times when things felt easier? What was happening then?'

We need to acknowledge and mark any positive response – 'That must have been good!' or we can use tonality 'Mm' so that the client, usually unconsciously, notices that the response has been acknowledged and reinforced.

We need to reflect back to the client when *they* change tense about their problems and positively reinforce this.

Sometimes it seems difficult to get the client to acknowledge that there have been any times when they have felt better, in which case it is often useful to ask when it has got worse. If it can change for the worse, it implies that it can also change for the better.

> Marie comes into surgery and sits down with a sigh, saying 'I feel so tired and low I don't think I can go on working. I have been feeling like this for months and it isn't getting any better – only worse'
>
> Her focus is on the depression and how bad she feels – your job is to direct her focus to times when she felt a bit better. 'You say things are getting worse . . . so how were they before? Are there days (or hours) when you feel a bit better? How do you feel then? What are you doing differently then?'

▶ Balancing validation and change

We need to balance validation of the client's feelings with directing their attention to where they want to go. This is why building rapport is so important. If the health professional jumps immediately into solution-oriented talk without the client feeling that their problems and emotions have been listened to and understood, then the therapeutic relationship will be damaged and the client will probably not be willing to work with you. But if health professionals themselves keep their focus on solutions then they can pick up whenever the client mentions a positive or an exception to the problem and begin to develop it. They can ask the kind of questions that can begin to lead the client towards a solution orientation and where they want to go.

1. **Change tense**

2. **Mention limited periods of time**

3. **Mark exceptions**

The difficulty is getting the balance between gathering a good history and associating the client into their problems, which entrenches them further. Asking for the 'Reader's Digest' version of their life story can be helpful.

One way I have found useful in taking a history from a client is to ask them to bring with them a sheet of paper upon which they have drawn their life line and upon which they have marked events that they felt have been significant. If the line is pencilled above the life line it indicates a positive feeling generated by the event, if it is below it indicates a negative feeling.

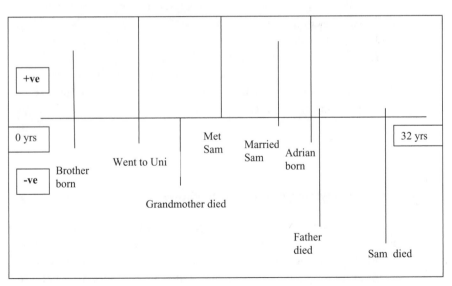

Figure 6.4 Positive and negative life events portrayed on a lifeline.

This can be a useful starting point for discussion and can give you clues as to a client's difficulties.

Listen for your client's metaphors, the way that they describe the problems that they are having. This will give you useful information and if you build and expand on your client's metaphors, they will be more meaningful and effective for that particular client, than any imagery and metaphors that you, the health professional, generate.

▶ 'What do you do already that helps?'

'What do you do already that helps?' is a question that should be asked whatever the emotional problem presented. Clients have strengths and resources that sometimes they are unaware that they are using and you can direct their attention to these.

> Mark presented with needle phobia and had bottled out at the last minute when having to have vaccinations for a business trip to the Far East. When asked what helped when he felt anxious on other occasions, he replied that he was a keen violinist and played his favourite music 'in his head' 'to keep calm'.
>
> Gillian came to see me because she had realised that her obsessive–compulsive disorder worsened significantly when she felt stressed and she wanted help with her levels of anxiety. On asking her what she did already that was helpful she replied 'I have a fish tank in my lounge and I sit on the settee next to it and swim with my fishes'. Using her imagination in this way helped her feel calmer.

▶ 'Is there anything else I need to know?'

Another question that I recommend using when the client has finished giving you their history is 'Is there anything else I need to know?' It is surprising how many clients take a deep breath at this point and then divulge information that is more important than any that has come before . . .

Sarah had given a history of depression stretching back over many years. She had had a fairly unremarkable childhood although she said that her father had been in the army and had been quite authoritarian. Her mother had worked hard and with three other children had not given Sarah a lot of attention and encouragement. She had been bullied at school and was glad to leave. She enjoyed her job as a clerical officer but had difficulty mixing and making friends. When asked if there was anything else I needed to know, she told me about her first boyfriend who had been killed in a motor bicycle accident and how she had had her most severe bout of depression after her grandmother had died. She had been very close to her grandmother and had lived with her on and off as a child. 'She was like my Mum, really'.

▶ Summary

HOW rather than why?

Imply change

■ Change tense

■ Mention limited periods of time

■ Mark exceptions

Obtain the 'Reader's Digest' version of their life story

What do you do already that helps?

Is there anything else I need to know?

Cognitive distortions

We measure our reality in words, we language our thoughts and often make the mistake of believing what we tell ourselves. But our perception is only one truth and is subject to many distortions, many of which we are unaware of until we stop and think about them.

There are many ways people distort their thinking and if we can bear these in mind when clients are telling us their problems, it can give us a way to help them towards a different perspective. After all isn't that what we want to do? The desired outcome of any psychological intervention is to help the client move from where they are now to where they want to be in the future, and to do that they need to see where they are going! One way of doing this is to help the client towards different perceptions of 'the problem'.

▶ I feel = I am

We have already mentioned one distortion – that of equating how one feels with one's identity. We need to be on the lookout for this and help clients understand that they are more than their current emotional state by leading them to notice exceptions and their own particular patterns. This can lead to connecting them to solution behaviours that can be re-enforced and practised.

I Feel = I Am

Julia comes into your surgery complaining of panic attacks. She tells you 'I've always been anxious. I think I was born that way! Mum always used to say I was a highly strung child'.

Explore times when she didn't feel anxious, especially those times when she expected to feel anxious and didn't or carried on regardless.

▶ Black and white thinking

One of the most popular of the ways we use to distort our perceptions is that of black and white thinking, of believing that something is all or nothing. 'I never do that' or 'I always feel anxious'. By gently challenging such assumptions, we can direct the client towards a realisation that maybe sometimes they don't react like that, that feelings and behaviour can be changed. One phrase I often use (thanks to Bill O'Hanlon) is 'I always do that, except when I don't!'

Children think very much in terms of black and white 'If you are not best friends then you must be an enemy'. Usually, as we grow older (?and wiser) we realise that most things are shades of grey. We begin to realise that most things in life lie on a continuum.

▶ Generalisation

In the same way we magnify, minimise or overgeneralise. If we leave words such as 'never' and 'always' unchallenged, then we have missed a golden opportunity to help our clients gain some insight into their emotional predicament.

Overgeneralisation

John, a father of three, has just been made redundant. He sits at home, feeling very depressed and says to his wife 'I'm a failure at *everything* I do. There's no point to *anything* – I might as well give up!'

Gwen is in the process of divorce. She tells her friend 'You can't trust people – they *always* let you down. I'll have to get used to being lonely – I'll *never* be able to have a relationship again.'

▶ Focus of attention

We all view the world through an emotional filter. If we are happy we shrug off adversity and notice all the positives, but if we are feeling depressed we only notice the negative side of events. We see whatever we need to see to confirm our current emotional state. This isn't something wrong – we all do it.

We are very good at focusing our attention on some things and not noticing others. Until I mention it, you are probably not aware, while you are reading this book, of how your left foot feels or the feel of your watchstrap on the skin of your wrist. They are still there sending sensory information to you but you were unaware of them consciously until you directed conscious attention to them.

One useful way of helping clients realise that they have this focus of attention is to ask them to look around the room and notice all the square or oblong shapes, pictures, windows, etc. and point them out to you. When they have done this ask them how many round-shaped objects they had noticed at the same time. Assuming your room has several of each, it can be a good way for them to learn experientially that they only notice what they focus their attention upon. We will talk more about focus of attention when we look specifically at anxiety and depression.

Stories are also a good way of making the point and I often tell clients a story that actually happened. Our medical centre is in an old building that housed the District Bank for many years while we rented the adjoining bank manager's house. When the bank decided to close its branch, we took over the entire building. The massive old front door and bank counter were left intact, together with the legend 'District Bank' in the stonework over the front door. Inside it was patently obvious, one would think, that this was a doctor's surgery. But one afternoon, about two years after the Bank had ceased to exist, a bank robber with a stocking mask held up our staff at gun point and demanded money. It took until he had counted to six before he realised that what our staff were telling him – that this was a doctor's surgery, no longer a bank – sank in and he ran out. He saw what he was expecting to see and it took some while before the reality sank in and changed his perception.

Our sense of time also gets distorted. When we feel anxious or depressed, it feels as if it has always been like this. We slip into all or nothing thinking again and discount anything that does not confirm our emotional state. Taking a negative comment at face value and not exploring it to find shades of grey or exceptions is a missed opportunity to help our clients learn a new perspective.

Emotional Filter

Judith had just returned from a week's holiday. Her husband had had too much to drink on a couple of nights and had embarrassed her in the hotel bar. When asked how her week had been she said 'We had an awful holiday – Jim got drunk in the bar and really showed me up!'

On further questioning the other five days and nights had been fine and she had enjoyed herself, swimming and dancing but she had negated that and spread the negative feeling over the whole holiday.

When working with someone, if when asking how the previous week or so has been, they tell you that they have had a bad week; request more information. Breaking the week down will often indicate that actually things had gone well for some time but that the client had forgotten this.

▶ Mind-reading

Another favourite distortion is mind-reading or crystal ball gazing! We think we know what someone is thinking or meaning by a particular behaviour or response. Unfortunately, we often get it wrong! If we do not challenge such assumptions in our clients, they continue to think that what they surmise is true. One needs to look for evidence to support or refute one's mind-reading. Could there be other explanations, other possibilities? Or should one learn to tolerate uncertainty – one of the most difficult things we can help our clients to do.

Mind-Reading

Ann sees four of her work colleagues talking. They stop when she approaches. She thinks to herself 'They were talking about me – they must have heard the boss shouting at me'.

This gives Ann a negative feeling but what other explanation could there be?

Perhaps they were planning a surprise for her 40th birthday?
Perhaps they weren't talking about her at all?
Perhaps Ann could ask?

We often say 'I can't do that' but what we need to encourage our clients to do is to explore the possibility 'What would happen if you did?'

If your client wants to gaze into a crystal ball, then encourage them not to see just one scenario (usually the worst one if they are depressed or anxious) but to see as many different possibilities as they can. Do not fall into the trap of believing that you, as the health professional, have a crystal ball! The catastrophic thinking of the anxious and depressed client may come true but it is only one of many possibilities and is it a good and resourceful way to live life focused on only this dire possibility?

Pessimists may have a more 'realistic' view of the world and optimists may distort reality, feeling that they have more control than they actually do and that more good events than bad happened (Alloy & Abramson, 1979). The depressed client may have a more realistic view of life but it doesn't seem to help them feel any happier!

Looking at possibilities and weighing probabilities is a skill that we can help clients use (see Chapter 11).

Crystal Ball Gazing

Kate's mother-in-law usually comes over for the day on Christmas Day. Kate resents the fact that she can't spend Christmas just with her husband and child but fears what her mother-in-law would say if she suggests that she comes round on Boxing Day.

Having looked at various possible responses, Kate plucked up courage to ask and was pleasantly surprised when her mother-in-law was really grateful because she didn't want to turn down an invitation from an old friend to stay with her but hadn't wanted to upset her daughter-in-law.

▶ Try, must and should

'Try' is another word to watch out for because it implies failure. If you 'try and get to sleep', the chances are you will fail. So when clients tell me that 'They'll try' and do the homework that we've decided upon, I ask them not to try, to either do it or not do it!

A common distortion that we need to be alert to is when we hear clients use the words 'must' and 'should'. Very often these are dictats they lay upon themselves or others that may not be appropriate. Would they feel better if they changed the 'musts' and 'shoulds' to 'prefer' or 'would like'? 'Musts' and 'shoulds' fuel anger better than anything else (see Chapter 13). Using 'prefer' or 'would like' in one's internal dialogue reduces the emotional temperature!

Must and Should

Tom comes back from work and sees the living room in a mess. He flies into a rage and sweeping the toys into a bin bag, shouts 'The children have got to learn! They must clear up their toys or I'll throw them away!'
Is this good for Tom or his children?

▶ Personalisation

Some clients tend to take blame even when inappropriate or feel that something is entirely their fault when anyone else can plainly see that it is not. They tend to take criticism personally rather than seeing it as directed at their behaviour (see Chapter 14). This personalisation is a key factor in depression and can often be seen in clients with low self-esteem. In these cases, the client needs to learn to 'take a step back' from the situation and look at it from an 'observer' viewpoint (see page 132).

Personalisation and Blame

Mary has made a mistake at work. Her manager is angry and shouts at her. Mary retreats to the toilet in tears thinking 'It's all my fault – I'm useless'.
Re-attribution of blame – look at the different factors influencing the outcome – is the manager having a bad day – maybe he has some other reason to be angry?

▶ Behaviour = identity

In the same way that a client can equate 'feeling' with 'being', they can also equate 'doing' with feeling and then with 'being'.

> ### I Do = I Feel = I Am
>
> Richard dropped an easy catch at an important cricket match and felt very embarrassed. 'I feel so stupid, I'm a fool' he tells his friend in the bar afterwards 'I don't know how I could have missed it!'
>
> Why does missing a catch = being a fool (identity)?

▶ Evidence

So it is very important to notice the language your client uses and begin to direct them to look at evidence for their way of thinking. Maybe they can ask other people's opinions or find some way of testing out their beliefs. Often people are much harder on themselves than on others – what would they think about someone in their situation? Would they think what they believe about themselves? We will talk later about perceptual positions (see Chapter 13) but putting yourself 'in someone else's shoes' is a very good way of beginning to change rigid perceptions.

▶ Cost-benefit analysis

Another good way of getting someone to think and evaluate their perception is to do a cost-benefit analysis by listing the advantages and disadvantages of a particular feeling for themselves either writing them down or doing it internally. For instance, if the bus is late, are you going to affect when the bus arrives by worrying about it? But is there something that you can do to mitigate the effects of the bus arriving late? Maybe ring someone and say that you have been delayed? Resolve to leave home earlier next time? Anxiety is useful but once you have learnt what is necessary it becomes a hindrance.

▶ Counselling 'swear words' needing a challenge

Always . . . except when you don't

Never . . . except when you do

Must . . . prefer

Should . . . would like

Try . . . do or not do

> ## Examples of phrases that need challenge or qualification to help your client begin to gain a different perspective

Why not match up the challenges with the phrases? More than one challenge may apply in each case. (Answers in Appendix VI on page 243)

Phrase	Challenges
1. 'People scare me'	(a) What would happen if you did / didn't?
2. 'He makes me feel so angry!'	
3. 'That was the worse time of all'	(b) Has there ever been a time when you didn't? What was different?
4. 'I handled that meeting badly'	
5. 'He is better than I am'	(c) In what way?
6. 'I must go to work'	(d) Who won't?
7. 'She just makes me feel bad'	(e) Always . . . all the time . . . every minute of every day?
8. 'I can't ask her out'	(f) How does it mean that?
9. 'They are out to get me'	(g) Why do you feel that?
10. 'That is not important'	(h) Where is your evidence for that?
11. 'They won't listen to me'	
12. 'She hurt me deeply'	(i) How does this seem to happen?
13. 'I can't fly'	(j) Who is?
14. 'I feel angry'	(k) Compared with what?
15. 'I can't say no'	(l) Worse than what?
16. 'She's always yelling at me; she hates me'	(m) What stops you from changing it?
17. 'He forgot my birthday; he obviously doesn't really love me'	(n) Can you think of any other reasons for someone to do this?
	(o) How specifically?
18. 'I never seem to do anything right'	(p) Better at/than what?
	(q) Never, ever?
19. 'You can't trust people'	(r) Who specifically?/Who says?
20. 'I always feel anxious'	(s) How would she know that?
21. 'I regret my decision'	(t) Can you think of any time when you can/did?
22. 'If she knew how much I liked him she wouldn't do that'	(u) What stops you?
	(v) About what? To whom?
23. 'He doesn't like me'	(z) What leads you to believe that?

▶ What are your favourite ways to distort your thinking?

How might you challenge these?

1. I feel bad and that I have not done well - therefore I am bad and a failure. I feel = I am and I do = I am

Separate doing, thinking and feeling from identity – you are more than. . . .

2. Black and white thinking – it's all or nothing

Look for shades of grey . . . maybe a failure can be viewed as a partial success if you have learnt from it?

3. Overgeneralisation – viewing one event as part of an unchanging pattern

Find exceptions to the pattern

4. Emotional filter – discounting positives, focusing on the negative

Write down the three best things you notice each day; mindfulness training

5. Mind-reading

Where is the evidence? Why not ask in order to check it out? Are you using double standards, believing that someone will think differently from how you would expect to react yourself?

6. Crystal ball gazing

Generate alternative possibilities . . . which are more probable?

7. Must/should/ought/have to – internal 'commands'

Change internal dialogue to 'prefer' and 'would like' . . . who is really doing the commanding and why?

8. Personalisation and blame – being very self-critical, taking all the blame when it was not entirely your fault; or alternatively blaming everyone else entirely

Acknowledge that there may be many influencing factors . . . have the attitude of a compassionate friend.

CHAPTER EIGHT

Seeding ideas

> Insanity is doing the same thing over and over again and expecting a different result.
>
> Albert Einstein

In this chapter, I would like to talk about some of the useful ideas and concepts that you can seed with your clients during a consultation. These ideas underpin brief psychological interventions and will lead towards the client altering their perceptions. They are not so much interventions themselves as the mindset one needs to develop in order to change and live one's live resourcefully.

Because metaphor is such a powerful tool, I will include some of the metaphors that I commonly use with clients. A picture speaks louder than words and if you can paint a verbal picture for your clients, drawing on their or your own experience, it will convey the message much more effectively (see Chapter 3).

► Cycles of thought, behaviour and feeling

We mentioned this previously but it is so important that it bears repeating. Take specific instances from the client's experience if you can and explore with the client what they were thinking, how those thoughts were linked to feelings and how their behavioural response gave rise to thoughts and feelings about those thoughts and behaviours.

Or take an instance such as waiting for someone who is late for an appointment. Imagine the thoughts they would have, the feelings each thought would generate and then the behaviour that would be likely to ensue. Then looking at the behaviour, explore whether that would generate other thoughts and feelings.

	Thought and internal images	Feeling	Behaviour
Daughter is late	She's been raped She's been in an accident She's dead	Anxiety++	Shouting at daughter when she returns
	I'm at her funeral	Sorrow	Tears

This catastrophising thinking leads to more feelings of terror and anxiety and when the daughter comes home these feelings will probably lead to anger as well as relief (anger here as a mask for helplessness) and a row ensue!

Change is inevitable

I challenge anyone to tell me one thing that never changes. One of the misperceptions of someone who is very depressed is that things will never change. I use metaphors such as 'I wonder if you can remember looking at a photograph album and seeing how over the years you changed from being a little girl (or boy), through being a teenager, to being an adult. You changed over time almost without realising it. You changed your hairstyle and you felt differently at different times in your life'. This would not be an appropriate metaphor for someone who had a very unhappy childhood – you need to know a little about the client you are talking to.

Another metaphor that I use is that of having clothes in ones wardrobe that you once really enjoyed wearing but that now you would not contemplate going out in. Metaphors for change abound in nature – you can use your imagination as appropriate.

Anxiety is learnt – for our protection

Clients often tell me that they think they were born anxious. If this were true then there would be little point in trying to change. People may be born with a tendency to have a more anxious or depressed character but it is only a small part of the whole. I often tell clients that as a toddler they were not anxious, they would run out into a busy road or touch something hot but they learnt to be fearful for their own safety and protection. Some of us just learnt it too well.

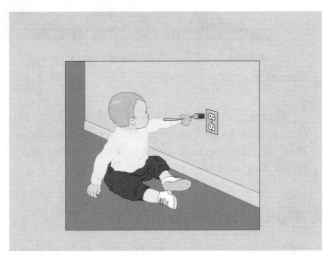

Figure 8.1   You are not born anxious

So anxiety has a protective value – up to a point. If I had no concern when I was asked to give a presentation, then I would not bother to prepare and probably do a poor job of it. Anxiety alerts us to possible problems and pitfalls, but once we have thought about what we need to do to avoid them, we no longer need the anxiety. If we keep our main focus on our goals rather than on the obstacles in the way, then we can find ways over or around them. If we focus just on the obstacles, we are brought to a standstill.

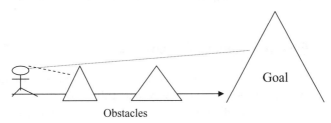

Figure 8.2   Do you focus on your goal or on possible obstacles?

Like most things in life anxiety can be seen as on a continuum – from unconcern to panic.

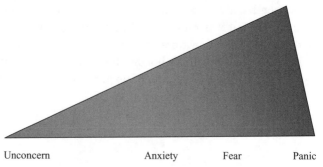

Unconcern   Anxiety   Fear   Panic

Figure 8.3   Anxiety continuum

Working with clients to help them achieve that balance is what good mental health care should be about. If anxiety is a 'learnt behaviour' or response then we can learn a better way of behaving or responding over time.

▶ Negative emotions are not 'bad'

Following on from this, another idea I like to get clients to understand is that negative emotions are not 'bad' of themselves. They are messages that can alert us to problems. It is only when we ignore the message that the negative feelings increase and expand. If we heed the whisper then we do not need to be shouted at. Anxiety is 'fear spread thinly' and fear is a message that we perceive danger in some way. Unhappiness means that we are discontented with how things are. Anger means that in some way our beliefs and values are being challenged or trampled on. Exploring emotions as messages can allow clients to begin to define the problems and then, with your help, hopefully begin to look at solutions. Once the client appreciates the message, they can learn ways of letting the feeling go.

▶ Positive intention of behaviours

Everything we do, we do at the time we do it because given how we are then it seems the best way to do things to get the desired outcome. This may be at an unconscious level – we may not be aware consciously of why we behaved or responded in a particular way. But I feel that it is very important to help clients begin to understand this. Many clients come in hating the part of themselves that behaves in a certain way and of course, like a child that is being rejected or ignored, it clamours more and more for attention. Accepting that this way of responding was perhaps all they could manage in time gone by, that it served them as well as it could, given their development and the context in which it occurred, means that they can begin to gain some self-acceptance. This does not mean that there are not things about themselves that they wish to change but self-acceptance is one of the building blocks to developing good self-esteem and assertiveness.

▶ We have all the resources we need

I firmly believe that we all have the resources, strengths and abilities within ourselves to make the changes we want – except when we don't!

In this latter case, one needs to think of ways that the client can begin to learn what they need to learn. Work with your client to devise some homework task that will help them to acquire the skills they need. Maybe they did have that skill sometime in the past or in a different context. In that case, you need to help them to remember this and to get them to really connect with that memory by getting them to relive it in their imagination as though it was happening in the present.

▶ All behaviour is patterned

Another concept that I find extremely useful to involve clients in is that nearly all our behaviour is patterned. When we learn a new skill, such as driving, it is a very conscious activity, but once learnt, we get into the car and just drive. This happens with all our activities – when did you last think consciously of how to walk or dress yourself?

It can be very useful to start interrupting some of our patterns. Suggest that your client start with something that is not important, maybe the way they get dressed or brush their teeth. Breaking a pattern a day helps you to build flexibility – and it can be fun! This kind of approach I often find useful with clients who have very rigid ways of thinking and behaving and with those with obsessive–compulsive disorder. With these latter, it is important not to get them to change the patterns that are central to their obsessiveness; that comes later in their own time, often without you needing to spell it out. The ripples spread outwards!

▶ All illness is psychosomatic

'Oh no it isn't' I imagine many people would say. I beg to differ. If I fall downstairs and break my leg, for a few split seconds it may be entirely physical (although some might ask why did I fall down then and not some other time!). Very shortly though, there will be an emotional response – 'How am I going to cope with work? How can I collect the children from school? This hurts!' – the psyche comes in and mixes with the soma! Alternatively, how can a mental illness not affect the body, given that our thoughts and emotions are mediated through neurotransmitters and chemicals within the body? The problem is with the overtones of the word 'psychosomatic' which has come to mean to some people that it is 'all in the mind' and therefore imaginary.

A pain is a pain even if the underpinnings may be mainly psychological in some cases rather than physical. Validating the client's symptom is of supreme importance, otherwise how can you possibly build rapport? But most clients will buy into the idea that how they feel emotionally does have an effect on how they feel physically and that can begin to give them the beginnings of control over at least the 'bothersomeness' of the symptom. There is an increasing body of evidence that shows that we can use our mind and our imagination to affect physical symptoms and parameters.

I sometimes tell clients of the time when I was organising a meeting and had a variety of forms that I had to fill out and distribute

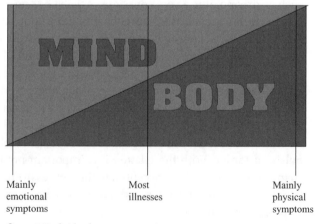

Mainly emotional symptoms   Most illnesses   Mainly physical symptoms

Figure 8.4 Mind / body representation

to various delegates at the meeting. Throughout the morning, I developed a throbbing headache and I decided to spend much of my lunch hour sorting and distributing the forms. As I handed over the last form, I casually and quite unconsciously remarked 'These forms give me a real headache!' As I heard myself say this, I realised that my headache had suddenly vanished as I had handed over the last form!

Most clients, I find, readily understand mind–body links once it is pointed out to them that they blush when embarrassed, perspire and go white when very anxious or fearful and most will have noticed that their symptoms are worse when they are 'stressed' or anxious.

▶ The past does not dictate the future

If you toss a coin and get heads six times in a row, it does not mean that it is any more likely than 50:50 to do so again on the seventh toss! Patterns may repeat themselves but if you can encourage the client to do something different, then the pattern will inevitably change. We will talk much more about this later. I tell clients that 'You are much more than your past, you are much more than the past events that have happened to you'. And, 'As you work to develop new ways of thinking and doing things, then, when you encounter situations similar to those in the past, you will react differently – things cannot be just the same because you understand things now that you didn't then'.

For those who enjoy computers, I use a computer analogy – it is as though you have added a new programme to your computer. The old one is still there – as a little icon that can be activated but you can minimise it and use the new programme to run your computer. Hopefully, you can help your client close the old programme down completely once you recognise that it is there running in the background. Maybe the computer is running slow (?depression) maybe it is unstable (having a sudden unexpected response to a situation, e.g. anger or fear).

Another metaphor I commonly use is Erickson's learning to walk metaphor (page 55). I find this is useful when clients have completed some work with me and have developed new ways of doing things because it helps them to view slipping back into old patterns as a temporary hiccup rather than as a failure. They are then much more likely to pick themselves up and try again.

▶ Solutions from the past

Many clients, when they feel stuck in some negative emotional state, forget that they achieved things in the past. It can be useful to explore whether they have encountered some problem in the past that mirrors in some way the problems they are having in the present. How did they deal with it? With hindsight (a wonderful tool) is there something that they would have done differently that would have been more helpful? Maybe they can utilise this in the future?

▶ Expectancy talk – presupposing change

If you work with clients and focus on problems all the time, you are much less likely to achieve solutions. If you work from the presupposition of change, you are much more likely to be successful. The client will begin to focus on how they want to be in the future and this helps their motivation. If you think they won't change, then this will be reflected in your non-verbal communications, if not in your words, and the power of suggestion can be used just as easily in a negative way as in the positive.

Sometimes our clients are afraid that their emotions will overwhelm them if they start to work with their problems. In this situation, I find talking about finding sluice gates and opening them so

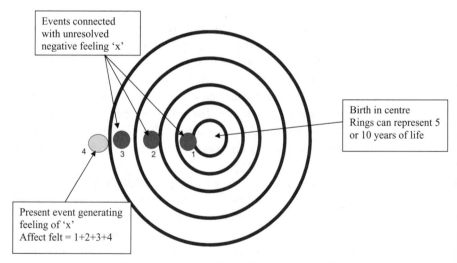

Figure 8.5   How unresolved feelings from the past influence the present

that the water level behind the dam can fall prior to work on it can be a help. In practice, this fear is more expectation than reality. Using imagery and metaphor can be a gentle and gradual way of allowing release of emotion.

Emotion generated by an incident in the present may be partly formed from similar unresolved emotional responses from the past. For instance, the loss of a pet may also reflect grief from loss of a loved one in the past that had not been worked through, so that the present emotional response seems inappropriately severe. Clients who show inappropriate anger, e.g. road rage, are often those with unresolved anger from the past.

Understanding this can give a great feeling of relief to someone who is worried and upset about the intensity of their emotional response.

▶ Summary

Useful ideas to seed with your client:

1. There is a continual cycle between our thoughts, our feelings and our behaviour.

2. Change is inevitable.

3. Anxiety is a learnt behaviour – therefore can be modified.

4. Negative emotions are not 'bad'.

5. Emotions can be regarded as messages.

6. All behaviour has a positive intention for the individual – at some level and at some time.

7. They have within themselves the resources needed for change.

8. All behaviour is patterned – changing a pattern changes the outcome.

9. All illness is psychosomatic – it has a physical and an emotional component.

10. The past does not dictate the future.

11. Always carry hope and expectancy.

CHAPTER NINE

Reframing

How we label things to ourselves generates emotion. By facilitating your client to see things from a different perspective, you can help them to reframe or re-label negative events or emotions. Often giving reassurance that the client is not 'going mad' may be helpful.

▶ Explanations

Explanations can be very useful. It is dangerous to assume that your client understands what is happening when they feel anxious. Many do understand the fight and flight response but it is worth checking this, as many do not. It is also worth pointing out that the mind cannot distinguish between vivid imaginings and reality when it comes to the adrenalin response – anxious thoughts build up anxiety response just as much as a threatening situation.

I often tell clients that if I injected them with adrenalin they would feel the physical effects for about 20 minutes – fast heartbeat, sweaty and light-headed, etc. However, normally what happens is that they notice the physical effect of the adrenalin they produce and then have an anxiety-provoking thought about this, which in turn produces more adrenalin and so on in a vicious cycle. This can go on for days on end, so is it any wonder that they feel tired all the time! Remember to perform thyroid function tests as an overactive thyroid may mimic an anxiety state.

Another response that is less commonly talked about is freezing, i.e. playing dead in the animal world. This is often not a good way to respond as the person is physically and emotionally 'stuck'!

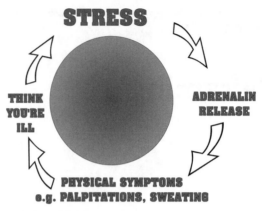

Figure. 9.1 Circles of fear

▶ Different perspectives

Reframing is what we do when we help the client gain a different perspective on their symptom or problem. We suggest a different context or frame to put around the problem. For instance: an elderly person's 'stubbornness' could be seen as the downside of a useful 'determination' that served them well throughout life. A teenager's 'rebelliousness' could be seen as a striving for 'independence'.

▶ Adrenalin states

Another idea that you could share with anxious clients is that we only have one adrenalin state – it is the labelling of it that makes it appear different. Get the client to describe how they feel physically when they get anxious; fast heartbeat and fast shallow breathing, sweaty, light-headed, nauseous, etc. Then ask them if they can remember 'having a crush' on someone when they were at school or if they can remember 'falling in love'. If they can do so, then ask them to remember how they felt when the object of their affections came into the room or spoke to them; fast heartbeat and fast shallow breathing, sweaty, light-headed, nauseous, etc. Of course, they then realise that the physical feelings were the same.

▶ Context and timing

Another way of reframing panic attacks is as an 'adrenalin burn' – for free! It is just in the wrong context. If the client lives near Blackpool

High adrenalin levels

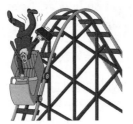

Rollercoaster - an adrenalin burn

For a shopper - a terrible panic attack

Figure 9.2   Panic attack or adrenalin burn?

or a theme park and enjoys roller coasters, then they'll know what you mean!

Some clients come in and think that they are 'going mad' because they think that there is no obvious reason for them to feel anxious or depressed. On further questioning about the previous year or two, you nearly always find that they have had all sorts of life events and problems to cope with. It is as though, having dealt with the crisis, they then have the time for the emotional response, later, when it is safe to do so. Realising this can often be helpful.

Anxiety states take time to build and also take effort and time to resolve.

> Once upon a time, a man was about to set out on a long journey across the dessert. He was loading up his camel with all the bags and baggages he was intending to take with him. He strapped on one bale after another, the poor camel was groaning under the weight. On went another blanket, another bale, another bag. He finally added one last water bottle and the camel collapsed, legs akimbo in the dessert sand. 'Alright' said the man, 'I'll take off that last water bottle'. Could the camel get up?

▶ Tolerating uncertainty

Sometimes one of the most important tasks we have is that of helping our clients tolerate uncertainty. If there were no uncertainty and we knew what would happen next, wouldn't life be boring?! Maybe we can help clients reframe their anxiety into anticipation – after all excitement and fear are both adrenalin states.

> Catherine suffered with flight phobia and after treatment decided to try going abroad on holiday. I suggested that if she had any apprehension, she should tell herself that she was 'excited' by going on holiday.

Many chronically anxious people avoid anything exhilarating or exciting and having them experience something exciting and notice how it feels can be very helpful as they become more used to realising that the feeling of adrenalin is not always bad.

▶ Labels and diagnoses

Diagnoses are often necessary for physical conditions so that causation and treatment can be accessed, but when it comes to our emotional health, they are often less than helpful.

People often like labels because it lends credence that what they are feeling is 'real' and acceptable. Sometimes a 'label' can mean that services can be accessed more readily. But more often, labels lead to restriction and anxiety.

No two people can ever really be sure that what they mean by a particular word is the same. Emotive words like pain, cancer and migraine carry meanings for us related to our past experience and vary from person to person. What is pain to me may be discomfort to you but no less real for all that.

> Sheila had been given the diagnosis of multiple sclerosis (MS) and came to see me two years later with severe depression and anxiety. Nothing had changed physically but her response to her symptoms had altered markedly with the label of MS. She had stopped many of her activities and begun to isolate herself socially. Upon exploring her feelings towards the diagnosis, I discovered that she had a picture of herself in a wheelchair every time she thought about having MS. Every time she got a twinge or a 'funny feeling' anywhere, she immediately keyed into this visual image. She had not taken on board what she had been told regarding the varying degrees of severity of MS at an emotional level, although she knew this at an intellectual level. One of the interventions she found helpful was for her to alter the image of the wheelchair into a comfortably upholstered armchair.

Clients have often told me that they understand why they have the feelings that they are experiencing but that knowing this doesn't seem to help them change the feelings. We all know that there are times when we tell ourselves that it is silly to feel the way we do but that this has little effect on our emotional state at the time. We can understand something intellectually but until we understand it emotionally, we do not change the way we feel.

▶ Right and left brain model

One model that can help clients understand why this is so involves thinking of the brain and its two cerebral hemispheres. The left hemisphere, which tends to process language and our critical, evaluative, logical thought processes, is that part of our mind or consciousness that we are generally most aware of in our day-to-day activity, our 'intellectual consciousness'.

The right side of our brain, which becomes more active as we relax or become deeply involved in some activity, is responsible for our visual and creative imagination. This part of our mind or our 'unconscious mind' constantly works in the background and controls all our bodily processes, such as our breathing and heart rate, and can also be seen as our 'emotional intelligence' as this is where we also process our feelings and emotions. This is, of course, merely a model, not the truth! The truth is that despite our increasing knowledge, we know very little and what we do think we know we cannot be certain about!

But as you begin to relax, become deeply absorbed in some activity or start to visualise, you begin to shift over to a 'right brain' mode of functioning. The critical, evaluative thought processes (predominantly a left brain or conscious operation) start to lessen and suggestions are more easily accepted. This is why hypnotic or visualisation techniques work so well with people, – they work with symbol and metaphor, which is the 'language' of the 'right brain' or of the 'unconscious', where we process emotion.

This shift in brain activity also occurs quite spontaneously throughout our day. Whenever we find ourselves gazing out of the window in a daydream; driving on 'auto-pilot', with no conscious recollection of the last few miles; whenever we become totally focused on an activity and start to lose awareness of our surroundings, we are predominantly in a 'right brain' state.

It is extremely useful to teach people how to access this state of mind, whenever they wish it; to bring it under their own conscious control, so that they can utilise it to help themselves achieve greater calmness and self-confidence.

I will describe how this approach can be used very effectively to help clients with anxiety and depression in Chapters 10 and 11.

It can be very helpful to have a folder in your consulting room with pictures similar to those in this chapter. A picture can explain and reinforce the ideas that you are trying to communicate to your clients.

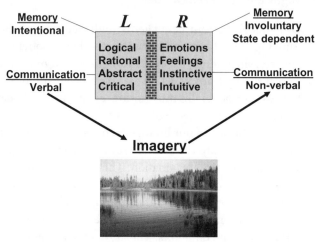

Figure 9.3   R/L brain model

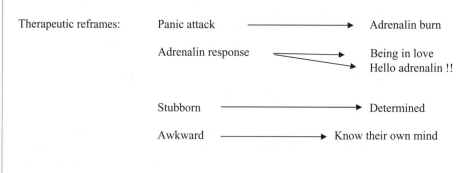

Therapeutic reframes:

Panic attack ⟶ Adrenalin burn

Adrenalin response ⟶ Being in love
Hello adrenalin !!

Stubborn ⟶ Determined

Awkward ⟶ Know their own mind

Temporal reframes:

I am depressed ⟶ While you **have been** feeling low….

When you **were** ….

Figure 9.4   Therapentic and temporal reframes.

▶ Summary

- Reframing: This means placing things in a different 'frame' or context, thereby encouraging a change in perception.

- All therapy could be regarded as reframing – helping the client to find a different perspective.

- Reframe anxiety into anticipation and excitement?

- Help clients to tolerate uncertainty.

- Labels and diagnoses can be useful so long as they are not restrictive.

- The right/left brain model can be usefully explained to clients.

CHAPTER TEN

Patterns: how? rather than why?

I am going to look at anxiety and depression together because I think that to split them into two separate conditions is fallacious. I feel, based on more than 30 years experience in general practice that anxiety and depressive symptoms always occur together in varying degrees.

We have talked already about how clients often take on their current emotional state at the level of identity and if your focus is entirely on the reasons *why* the client is depressed or anxious, it will often not lead you very far in helping the client to change how they feel.

How do you do it?

Asking *how* they depress themselves or *how* they do anxiety can give you useful insights into how they could do it differently. This has to be done in rapport and preferably after you have seeded some of the ideas we have already mentioned in this book.

You need to get the client to be very specific. What behaviour are they doing? What pictures are they seeing in their mind's eye? What are they telling themselves or thinking about? Get them to imagine teaching you how to do depression or anxiety in the way that they are. How do they know what kind of a day it is going to be when they first wake up?

Other useful information can be gathered by asking clients what they do differently when they are not feeling depressed or anxious. What happens on the days when they feel a bit better?

This kind of investigation I often suggest as homework, to be written down and brought to the next consultation. I suggest that they become their own detective.

▶ Smoke alarm

Once the client is beginning to think along these lines, it is often useful to get them to recognise the first step on the path to feeling depressed or anxious. This can then be their 'smoke alarm', alerting them that some intervention is needed or they will spiral down becoming more and more depressed or anxious. Telling them your own smoke alarm can be helpful as an example. Mine is a feeling of wanting to go for a long, solitary walk on the hills or a queasy feeling in my stomach!

Once you have elicited some sort of a pattern then suggest that the client has a go at doing something different. Making one change in the pattern can often lead to substantial changes in the client's emotional state.

For instance, I remember one client I was working with who used to walk her dog in the park every day. I set her the task of noticing the differences between when she felt bad and when she felt better. One of the differences she noticed was that on a bad day she walked slowly and didn't look at anyone or notice her surroundings. On a good day, she walked briskly and looked around herself more. I suggested that now she had noticed this difference, she could perhaps try walking briskly and looking around on the days she felt bad and notice what happened.

Another client noticed that on not-so-good days she stayed in bed a lot longer and didn't bother to shower; so she changed her pattern by making sure she had a shower when she got up on these not-so-good days.

Find the pattern – and then change it in some way.

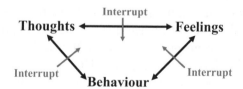

Figure 10.1   You can interrupt the pattern at any point

When someone is extremely depressed or anxious, they feel that they have no control and suggesting that they could do one thing that is not too demanding will begin to give them back that control. It is important that the client will actually do as you suggest so keep your suggestions simple.

▶ When someone is drowning, it is not the time to offer them a swimming lesson

I find a useful intervention when someone is extremely distressed is to teach them a breathing exercise. This can be done in a 5- or 10-minute consultation in surgery – it does not take long. Very commonly, when a client comes to see you and has been feeling very upset and anxious for a while, suggesting that they sit down and do a relaxation technique will be impossible for them.

However, even those who are not hyperventilating are often breathing fast and shallowly and teaching slower diaphragmatic breathing can be a very useful way of helping them to relax without focusing on *trying* to relax. Anxiety is linked to rapid breathing using the upper chest muscles and learning a technique that encourages diaphragmatic breathing will help clients feel calmer and change their focus of attention to their breathing rather than on their anxiety.

Breathing Exercise (1) – place your hands flat on either side of your chest, with your thumbs just below the lower ribs – focus your attention on your hands and imagine the air flowing in and out through your fingers – maybe imagining the air as a colour, maybe the colour of calm. Continue doing this for several minutes. When you have got used to doing this, they can then start to do it without actually putting their hands in position, just focusing their attention there. I also suggest that they count as they breathe. Breathe in for, say a count of 3, hold for a count of 3 and then breathe out for a count of 4.

Increase the count as is comfortable for them but breathing out should always be one count more than the time they breathe in and the time they hold. This counting pattern helps to hold their attention and will also stop hyperventilation. If you only teach diaphragmatic breathing, then the danger is that the client who hyperventilates will continue to do so, only even more effectively!

I would suggest that clients do this exercise every hour or two for a couple of minutes, or at least twice a day for five minutes, depending on the circumstances. They can then do the exercise whenever they feel themselves getting anxious. This will do two things. They will start to use the diaphragm when they breathe and this breathing pattern will not only help them feel calmer, but it will also focus their attention away from the anxiety. Although this technique can be useful for someone who is very distressed, it is also useful to teach to someone who is becoming anxious, as they will find it easier to practise when they are not too panicky.

Another exercise I commonly teach to anxious clients in a surgery consultation is this.

Breathing Exercise (2) – simply close eyes and watch your breathing, which is always with you – become aware of the rise and fall of your chest, of the flow in and out of your breath. Don't try and change it in any way, just be aware of your breathing. Follow the flow of air in and out through your nose and notice the slight temperature difference between the air you breathe in, which is slightly cooler than the air you breathe out, because the air you breathe out has been warmed by its journey through your lungs. Just <u>be</u> with your breathing – you don't have to *do* anything at all. If a stray thought comes into your head, let it flow out again, you don't need to follow it, just focus back on the rise and fall of your chest, the flow of air in and out. If part of you feels uncomfortable, then maybe direct your out-breath into that part. Letting go with each outgoing breath. After a few minutes, begin to focus on that split second when your in-breath becomes your out-breath, and your out-breath becomes your in-breath. . . . You could then visualise a patch of blue sky with a great bird flying – the wings beating in time with your breathing or take yourself in imagination to a calm, relaxing place and really be there, seeing, hearing, smelling and feeling the place you have chosen. Some people like to imagine 'the colour of calmness' flowing in with each in-breath and flowing around their body with each out-breath.

This is a self-hypnotic technique that I find most clients really like. It is focusing their attention on something that is always with them, their breathing; and most importantly, it is not trying to change anything. Because, by focusing attention and visualising, they are automatically entering a 'right-brained' state, they will start to relax. Focusing in this way will often be more successful in helping the anxious client to relax than a 'normal' relaxation technique where you consciously aim to relax – here you don't *try* to change anything – just be. 'Trying' nearly always implies failure! It is NOT, however, a good technique to teach a client who is obsessing about their breathing.

► Physical tension

In the same way as clients who are anxious and depressed tend to have a particular breathing pattern, they also commonly complain of various aches and pains. I sometimes suggest that the client clenches their fist hard while we are talking and then after a few minutes ask them to relax it and tell me how it feels. Of course it will feel quite uncomfortable and this can help them to understand experientially that holding muscles tense, which we all do especially when anxious, can lead to chest pains, headaches and other muscular aches and pains. I then suggest that they start getting used to doing a body scan whenever they are perhaps sat down watching TV or standing at the sink washing up. Doing this often throughout the day will help it to become second nature.

Body Scan – take a moment or two to mentally run over your body and check whether you are holding any muscles tight – then let go the unnecessary muscle tension consciously and deliberately on an out-breath.

► Body language

The way we hold our body, or our body language, is very linked to our emotional state; it has developed this link over years. I sometimes get clients to stand up, hunch their shoulders and look down at the floor. While holding that position, I ask them to feel confident. I then ask them to stand to attention, put their shoulders back, look up and notice how different that feels. Try to feel harassed and anxious while in this position and they will find it much harder to do because this body posture has been linked to feelings of confidence throughout their life. By doing this simple experiment, they can feel the effect of a positive link they have already built up over so many years that it is now a part of their physiology.

A depressed client will tend to look down as they ruminate inside so suggesting that your depressed client goes for a 30-minute walk every day and looks at the treetops or the chimney pots will help them to begin to shift. Looking up will help them to feel better and of course the physical exercise will help use up a little of that adrenalin.

The link between our body language and our emotional state is also present in our smile. Try smiling at yourself in the mirror when you feel low and after a few moments notice how your mood lifts a little.

▶ **Revivification**

Another very useful tool is that of revivification. This simply means getting the client to re-experience, as vividly as they can, some time and place where they felt relaxed and calm. Once the right kind of memory has come to mind, they go back into it, seeing what they saw, hearing what they heard, feeling what they felt (see Chapter 12 on anchors).

If someone is very anxious, I find it useful to suggest that they go back and re-experience some physical activity (such as swimming, cycling, horse riding) and then gradually, in their own time, slow it down until they are floating or dismounted maybe under some trees, depending on the activity they have chosen. The adrenalin that they have in their bodies when feeling anxious will match the physiological state of the activity they are imagining. Swimming is a good one because they can eventually imagine floating, completely supported by the water, with a slight movement rocking them gently. By visualising in this way, they are automatically going to begin to relax as they go into more of a right-brained state – but they don't need to 'try' and relax.

> You *can* be relaxed and you *don't have to* be relaxed.
>
> Bill O'Hanlon

▶ **Summary**

- Find out the pattern of your client's problem – then get them to make a change.

- Determine the client's smoke alarm – helps them to be aware of the start of a relapse.

- Interrupt thoughts – see chapter on Cognitive Distortions.

- Interrupt feelings – use imagination to revivify a pleasant time, mindfulness training.

- Interrupt behaviour – body scan, breathing exercises.

CHAPTER ELEVEN

What if?

> Worry is interest paid on something that may never happen.

Any anxious or depressed client will be focusing their attention either on the past or the future. If the past they will be ruminating on past traumatic events, if the future they will be painting a black future, if they see one at all; or worrying about what will go wrong. Catastrophic thinking is a hallmark of the anxious client. If this way of thinking was helping them identify where things went wrong in the past so that they could take steps to help in the future then this would be useful, but this is rarely the case. Such a focus of attention tends only to intensify the negative feeling.

▶ Catastrophic thinking

'What if' scenarios and the associated fears are often less frightening if 'taken out of the bag' and examined . . . take the feared scenario to its worst conclusion – that is only one possibility – what are the others? How would you deal, practically speaking, with the worst-case scenario? Are there some positive possibilities? – what would turn a possibility into a probability? Writing down other possibilities often helps to make them more specific and concrete. If they really believe that worst-case scenario do they do so sufficiently to bet on it with a fiver? They have to actually pay the fiver to charity if they are wrong! I have sometimes used this most effectively!

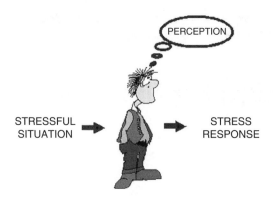

PERCEPTION

STRESSFUL
SITUATION

STRESS
RESPONSE

Figure 11.1

1. **REMOVE THE STRESSOR** using planning, prioritisation, delegation or ditch it.

2. **CHANGE THE PERCEPTION** using visualisation and challenging thoughts.

3. **CONTROL THE STRESS RESPONSE** using relaxation and imagery.

▶ Rumination

Clients who continually ruminate on their worries need to break into the cycle. Thought-stopping techniques are useful to teach clients like this. When they recognise that they are on the 'worry wheel', they shout 'stop' internally and visualise a 'stop' sign, or they could begin to count backwards, maybe in sevens, from three hundred, or they could snap a rubber band that they could keep on their wrist.

You cannot stop thinking of a pink elephant just by telling yourself to – but you can think of an orange giraffe instead! Get the client to interrupt the cycle and consciously and deliberately think of something else.

I am a great believer in writing things down because it forces clients to be specific and it gives them a distance from their problems so that it is easier to deal with them. I find this especially useful for those clients who lie in bed worrying. I suggest that they have a paper and pencil by their bed and write down whatever they start to worry about and then do a relaxation technique. They won't forget because they have written it down so they don't need to keep it in their head and they can address the problem in the morning.

▶ Worry time

This is also useful to do during the day if they keep a notebook in their pocket and they can then do a breathing exercise, go for a walk or some other activity. They then allocate half an hour (or longer) 'worry time' each day to look at what they have written down and review it.

I ask the client to break the worry down if at all possible. For instance, a large issue such as looking after an ill relative is too global. By breaking it down into its components such as doing their shopping, dealing with continual telephone calls, looking after their nutritional intake, sorting out financial problems, makes it much more accessible. Each item can then be looked at in turn and various questions can then be asked to help get things more in perspective.

Is it actually their problem or is it really some else's responsibility? If it is their problem, then can they do anything about it? Can they delegate part of it? Ask for help? Can they do things differently in some way that will help them feel better? Can they imagine putting it in a different time perspective – will it still be important in a year–10 years – in the history of the universe?

> **Break problems down**
> **Then use the three questions:**
>
> **Is it my problem?**
> **Can I do something about it?**
> **Will it still be important in 10 years?**

Sometimes I ask clients to bring in their list and we go through it together. Often simple changes can really make a difference.

Some of us are larks and are at our best in the morning but others are owls and find it easier to work in the evening. Knowing when you are at your best (premium time) is useful because you can plan to do something more taxing then and leave easier things to other times. It may be that the client needs to have a protected time to do a particular task and it is important that they plan this and tell those around that they do not wish to be disturbed. If they fail to do this, then interruptions are likely to occur causing irritation and rising stress levels.

▶ Plan and prioritise

Often when we feel pressured we tend to feel that everything has to be done at once and it all gets too much. We then either end up doing nothing or feeling bad about all the things we haven't yet done.

Some clients find it useful if they feel overwhelmed to sit down and compile a list of tasks that need doing. These then need to be looked at – are they really essential? If, after some thought, they decide a thing has to be done, then they need to decide how urgent it is. If it has high priority then they need to motivate themselves to do it (see Chapter 5 on goal setting). Set themselves the task of doing something specific and easily achievable that needs doing each day – then, once that has been done, anything else they do that day can be seen as a bonus.

▶ Delegation

Can they perhaps get someone else to take on some of their load? Delegation can be difficult as people often feel they could do it quicker and better than the other person. But we learn by doing things ourselves and maybe they need to let that other person learn to do things as well as they do – even if they make mistakes at first. After all, if we didn't make mistakes, how would we improve and get better?

THE THREE 'D's	THE THREE 'P's
DITCH IT	PLAN
DELEGATE IT	PRIORITISE
DO IT	PREMIUM TIME

▶ Time for self

Suggesting that clients make sure that they write in some breaks to their day, especially at lunchtime, is also very important. Someone who is anxious will feel overwhelmed and time pressured and will begin to cut down on breaks and leisure activities at just the time when they really need them. They will find that they actually work better if they make sure to take the breaks they need. It is not 'cost-effective' to run your car at 70 mph all the time. It is false economy to think you can work hard, all day, every day, without breaks. One may be able to do this for short periods but eventually it catches up with one.

It is a very good idea to take a 5- or 10-minute break in the middle of the morning and the afternoon, maybe to practise a relaxation technique, to have a short walk, or simply to sit down and have a cup of tea. We need to encourage our clients never to miss a lunch break; they shouldn't just snatch a sandwich while they work. They should have at least half an hour and sit down to eat, preferably away from their workplace. If they feel they can't do this, then they are working too hard and probably inefficiently. Encourage them to make some changes that ensure they can take a lunch break. They will work much more effectively and efficiently.

Encourage your clients to plan for some leisure time each week. If they don't actually plan their leisure activities, then it is very easy for the time to be swallowed up by something else.

Frequently, I use a metaphor that I heard from a colleague. When an architect designs a house, he makes sure that he builds good drains so that whatever rain or snow falls, it drains away without damaging the house. We all need to build our own drains, whether that relates to doing something physically active or something creative.

Guilt feelings about taking time out for oneself are common and I counter this by asking my clients whether they run their car without ever taking it to the garage or getting a service? When someone is having problems, their feelings impinge on everyone around them whether at work or at home. Taking time out for oneself is therefore not 'being selfish' but will help everyone if it helps the client to feel better. Ask the client to imagine stepping into the shoes of people around them and notice how they would think about it (perceptual positions). They will work much more effectively if they have taken time to recharge.

> It's hard to see the spot you are standing on – unless you move off it!

▶ Setting and achieving goals

A depressed and anxious client will feel it a great effort to do anything at all and often will feel overwhelmed and a failure. This, of course, confirms and feeds into their negative state. The feeling that there is so much they should do and haven't done only feeds feelings of despondency and anxiety. But tomorrow hasn't happened yet – what they do today can start to define tomorrow. So setting one goal a day and achieving it is the key here. I ask clients to write down each evening the one thing they are going to do the next day. This must be something that is relatively easily accomplished such as reading one chapter of a book, washing the pots, going for half-an-hour walk. When they have done it they cross it off their list and feel good about it. Having congratulated themselves on achieving one goal, anything else they achieve that day is a bonus that they can feel good about. Beware when clients start to set multiple or very large goals – it is important to emphasise to them that small steps are easier to take than a giant leap and they get to the same place in the end. One step at a time may seem unadventurous but will tend to be more successful in the long run.

> **Tomorrow hasn't happened yet**
>
> **Set one goal a day**
>
> **Everest was climbed by placing one foot in front of another – but it helps if you have a map**

▶ Focus of attention

Clients with high levels of anxiety or depression do not notice the present. And this is a shame because today very soon becomes yesterday and tomorrow becomes today. If clients are always focused on the negative then they never notice the things that could help them to feel better. Helping clients change this focus of attention is important.

▶ The three best things

I often suggest to clients with depression that they keep a notepad in their pocket and note down the three best things that they notice during the day. This could be the warmth of their shower in the morning, the taste or smell of something they ate or drank, something they saw, a flower or a smile. This begins to get a depressed person to shift their focus of attention from the negative and helps them to shift from a focus on the past or the future to the present. At the end of a week they will have 21 good things that they can reflect upon. Sometimes families who eat dinner together can make this a game where around the table they all tell in turn the three best things they noticed during the day. You don't need to be depressed to benefit from this!

Taking a little time each day to do a self-hypnotic technique can begin to help clients reduce their anxiety levels and the use of imagery for positive suggestion is a skill I teach many of my clients.

▶ Using imagination to help self-hypnosis and imagery

There are many ways for clients to use to do self-hypnosis. Apart from the breathing exercises and revivification already described, I sometimes teach a progressive muscular relaxation technique. This involves the client closing their eyes and allowing a feeling of comfort and maybe a colour flow down from the top of their head as they focus on each part of their body in turn. As they feel more and more comfortable, any tension can drain out of their feet into the floor. If one concentrates more on comfort than relaxation, it often works better. After all, you can be relaxed and you don't have to be relaxed. I then suggest that they take themselves in their imagination to a safe, calm, happy place, real or imaginary, and enjoy it.

If you wish to learn more of these techniques, then I suggest that you go on a basic training course in hypnosis where you can practise these techniques both for yourself and your clients.

It is a good idea to suggest that when clients do self-hypnosis they tell themselves how long they intend to be relaxing for, so that they get an internal nudge when to re-alert, as it is common to get time distortion. It goes without saying that one should not encourage clients to access trance states when driving or where it would be unsafe to do so.

Special place imagery

I like to get clients that I am working with develop imagery of a calm, relaxing, special place for themselves. The imagery that comes from their unconscious mind is going to be much more powerful for them than anything I can suggest. I set it up beforehand by talking about the kind of place they might find, inside or outside, real or imaginary and then ask that their conscious mind just wonders what will 'pop up' into their mind's eye when they are ready to go there.

Using imagery while in a right-brained or relaxed state to get rid of negative feelings can be helpful. Maybe before the client goes to their special place they could imagine a rubbish chute or a bonfire where they can throw away their anxious feelings or their frustration. Equally important is the use of imagery to focus on the positive feelings the client wants instead. Picking up a flower or a pebble from their special place that represents calmness or confidence and imagining bringing it back with them can be a way of giving themselves positive suggestion. Alternatively, seeing themselves the way they want to be in their special place and stepping into the image (see the following chapter) can be a powerful way of giving positive suggestion.

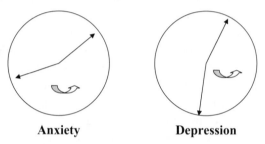

Anxiety   **Depression**

Figure 11.2   Control centre imagery

I sometimes suggest that clients should visualise their 'control centre' and look for the controls for anxiety and depression. Having seen what level they are set on (0–10 scale), they can then start to change them if they wish to. This is yet another way of using imagery for suggestion and can be surprisingly effective.

Clients suffering from anxiety or depression almost invariably suffer from tiredness all the time (TATT) and giving themselves suggestions of energy such as imagining being under a waterfall, absorbing the energy from the sun, or finding their own way of connecting with feelings of energy can be very effective.

Five-step self-hypnotic technique

(1) Sit or lie yourself down comfortably and take a deep breath in. As you breath out slowly, count to three in your head . . . '1 .. let your eyelids feel heavy, 2 .. let them close, 3 .. let that feeling of complete relaxation spread all over you'.

(2) Allow your body to relax bit by bit, maybe feeling heavy and comfortable, maybe imagine breathing in a colour that fills every part

of you as you relax, focusing on your breathing and letting the tension drain away with each outgoing breath . . .

(3) Use imagery to deepen your state of relaxation, for example going down stairs step by step, watching a balloon disappear into the distance, as you become deeper and deeper relaxed . . .

(4) Go to your own special place, real or imaginary, and enjoy it, remembering to use imagery to throw away negative feelings and give yourself some simple positive suggestions.

(5) When it is time to return to the here and now . . . count down from 5 to 1, opening your eyes and feeling wide awake and alert on the count of 1.

Some useful imagery

(a) Imagine walking down some steps to a bridge over a river or stream and stopping halfway over to get rid of any unwanted negative thoughts or feelings into the water and watch them being washed away. One can imagine throwing in a leaf or a stick symbolising the unwanted emotion. As you watch this being carried downstream and eventually out of sight, you can feel happy to be rid of the unwanted thing.

(b) You could use the imagery of a small, still pool that represents your 'pool of internal resources'.

. . . As you sit and gaze at the water, you notice that on the bottom of the pool are various stones and pebbles. These represent all the strengths and resources you already have, and you can feel pleased and encouraged as your unconscious mind identifies each resource, even though your conscious mind may not know what they are. Some you may have forgotten about, and others you may not even know you have, yet. Around the edge of your pool are various stones that represent other positive feelings or resources or those that you may want even more of . . .

Pick up a stone that represents 'x' (your unconscious mind will let you know which stone is the right one). Study it carefully, noticing its shape, texture, colour, and weight . . . then drop it gently into your pool, watching it drift down through the clear water to settle safely and securely on the bottom.

When you are ready, make connection with your pool in some way; maybe dabbling your hands and feet in the water, maybe swimming in it, and become fully in touch with all those resources within you . . .

Relaxation tapes can sometimes be useful but I prefer to encourage my clients not to rely on a tape as most people are not prepared to spend 30–40 minutes a day doing a relaxation technique. I suggest 10 minutes once a day is the minimum time needed to become reasonably proficient in self-hypnosis over three to four weeks and this is achievable by most with a bit of encouragement.

It is a good idea to suggest that clients tell themselves how long they are going to do their self-hypnosis for before they start so that their unconscious mind gives them a mental nudge when it is time to reorient back to the here and now. Remember also that any relaxation or hypnotic technique can lead into sleep, so if someone is overtired then setting an alarm clock may be useful! Although one can alert immediately if necessary, in an emergency, it is usually nicer to gradually reorient, especially if someone has become very deeply relaxed. Occasionally, if someone alerts too quickly, they can experience a slight headache. This is easily treated – go back into self-hypnosis and reorient more slowly. If you are intending teaching self-hypnosis to your clients, it really does pay to go on a basic hypnosis training course where you can practise in a safe, supportive environment.

The reset button

I suggest that if my client is very busy that they take half a minute now and again to recharge themselves. This exercise can be done frequently and, with practice, very quickly. It can be done anywhere, even in a busy office, as they don't need to close their eyes. The client can rest their chin on their hand and stare at the tip of their pen on the paper. With eyes open, I suggest that they focus on a suitable point and take a deep breath in. As they breathe out, they allow their body to relax and picture their special place. They imagine really being there and when they have hold of their symbol for calmness, they bring their focus back to the here and now, feeling refreshed. This acts rather like the 'reset' button on a computer and if done regularly can be effective in managing stress levels.

Mindfulness

If someone is very anxious, they will be focused worrying on the future, if depressed they will be ruminating on the past. In both cases, ways of connecting the person with their current sensory experience in a non-judgmental way (mindfulness) are very helpful. Encourage your client to every now and then really notice what they are doing, whether it is dinking a cup of coffee or washing their hands. Ask them to pay attention to the smell, the feel of the cup against their lip, the warmth and the flavour as they swallow; the feeling of the water on their skin, the smell and silkiness of the soap and the feel as they move one hand over the other. As they begin to notice the sensory information they are receiving, they become more connected to 'now'. Doing this on and off throughout the day can help change how people feel as they break into the patterns of their ruminations.

Mindfullness training can be very effective in helping people with emotional problems because they learn to 'take a step back' and observe without evaluation or judgement. Just sitting quietly and observing what you can hear, and then just being with your breathing as in the exercise on page 102 for a few minutes can be a useful step in helping the anxious client.

One metaphor I use is that the client needs to step out of the stream onto the bank so that they can just watch the stream as it flows by. Any thoughts or feelings that arise can just flow by in the stream.

▶ Scheduling

Any of the aforementioned self-hypnotic or relaxation techniques will benefit someone if done regularly. Discussing when the client could schedule doing this is important otherwise the temptation is to put it off, and with the feelings of fatigue and poor motivation that abound in anxiety and depression, it is quite likely that it will not become part of their day. Sometimes it can be very difficult to find a place where one can be undisturbed and stopping the car on the way home from work, locking the doors and taking five minutes out; or doing it in the bathroom may be the only way.

If at a follow-up consultation the client has not done their practice as they had said that they would, you need to help the client explore why they found it difficult and what got in the way.

▶ Summary

Catastrophisation . . . how would you cope practically with the imagined scenario? This is only one possibility – what are others? Which are more probable?

Rumination:

1. Thought stopping – interrupt thought cycle in some way

2. Write down the worry

3. Break it down into components if it is too global and vague

4. Question . . . is it my problem? Can I do something about it?

5. Temporal reframe . . . will it still be important in 10 years time?

Time management:

1. Plan – write them down

2. Prioritise – don't try to do too much all at once – one goal at a time

3. Remember to congratulate yourself when a goal is achieved

4. Take breaks regularly – to do exercise or something creative

Mindfullness:

1. Depression focuses on the past and anxiety on the future; both miss the 'now' – practise being in the present, noticing what you see, hear, smell, taste, feel, without judgement.

2. Write down the three best things noticed each day.

Self-hypnosis:

1. Reduces sympathetic activity (adrenalin)

2. Enhances effectiveness of suggestion

3. Accesses mind/body links

Imagery:

1. A calm, tranquil, safe, happy place – real or imaginary

2. Ways to discard negative feelings and symptoms – rubbish chute, bonfire, clouds and so on

3. Ways to give positive suggestion – symbolic imagery, control centres and associating with desired goal

CHAPTER TWELVE

Anchors and anchoring

> You can only have one thought at a time, so why not make it a good one?

We all know that smells, sounds, or seeing something can trigger memories. When we recall an event, we also re-experience some of the feeling associated with it. This fact is utilised in supermarkets when they waft the smell of fresh coffee or baking bread around to encourage us to feel good and buy more. For someone with a spider phobia the sight of a spider creates a link to some time when they associated a strong feeling of fear with seeing a spider and they instantly panic, even if they have no conscious recollection of where the fear came from. The sight of a spider acted like a 'hot button' to fear. You can help your clients create 'hot buttons' to good feelings such as confidence or calmness.

We all have inbuilt links related to our body language that have built up over time. As described on page 103, body posture is linked to feeling. To demonstrate this, I ask a client to stand with shoulders hunched and eyes cast down. While keeping this body position, I ask them to feel confident. Of course, this is very difficult in this position and usually we end up laughing at the impossibility of it. Once having straightened up, with shoulders back and eyes up, it is a very different 'feel'. A smile is another; where the tension in particular muscle groups involved in a smile has been linked over time with usage to happy feelings.

One can use concrete objects as links or triggers, such as pebbles or pictures, as in the following examples. I tell clients my own story of a beautiful plant I had been given that flowered and then started to die. I placed it in my back porch where I keep plants that are on their last legs. After some weeks, to my surprise, it started to flower again with beautiful purple velvety blooms. I was about to put it back on a window sill in the house when I thought 'No I will leave it here and it will give me a little burst of pleasure each time I see it when I go in and out.' So I did, and it still reminds me of beauty every time I pass it.

Case 2: Maureen

Maureen told me that she had several years ago gained her glider's license. She became quite animated while telling me about this and it was obviously a good resource for her, helping her to feel more confident and competent. I asked where she kept the photo of herself standing by the glider that she had described. She replied that it was in a drawer somewhere. I suggested that she find it and hang it somewhere where she would see it and remember and access the good feelings associated with it.

At her next visit, she told me that she had hung it in the hall and that she had noticed the good feelings she had each time she looked at it when passing by.

Case 3: Amy

Amy came in and started telling me about a walk she had had around our local reservoir. She was very proud of herself for having achieved this and she described her walk with great animation and enjoyment. I had a bowl of pebbles on my window sill and she remarked that some of them were just like a smaller version of the stones she had seen at the water's edge. I suggested that she choose one of my pebbles and let it be a reminder to her of the good time she had had. When she squeezed it in her hand she would be able to step into some of the good feelings that she had associated with her outing. She kept her pebble with her and often used it to remind herself that she could feel calm and confident.

The only problem with using concrete objects such as these is if they become broken or mislaid, but hopefully by this time the client will have other strategies and ways of helping themselves.

Music or sound can be used effectively to help access calmness or confidence. Some clients like to have pieces of music that they can play either in reality or in their imagination to access these feelings. The sound of waves on a seashore or the sound of running water are popular auditory links to calmness.

In the same way as certain external stimuli become associated with past experiences (thus recalling the past experience), one can DELIBERATELY ASSOCIATE a stimulus to the memory of a past experience.

Once this association has taken place, one can then trigger the memory of that experience at will together with the corresponding emotion that is attached to it. Often one will not recall the event but just get the feeling, as with the spider phobia example above.

By deliberately inserting some specific new stimulus while a person is fully in touch or reliving an experience, that new stimulus then becomes associated with the recalled experience. The new stimulus could be a touch, a sound or a visual image.

Reintroducing the same exact stimulus brings back into consciousness the feelings of the recalled experience. This procedure is known as *Anchoring* and the inserted stimulus is referred to as the *Anchor*.

The first step is to get the client to revivify or re-experience a time when they felt whatever the emotion is that they are after. This could be a time when they were being confident, in control, happy, exhilarated, or alternatively, it could be when they were feeling very calm and relaxed.

Notice that these two states are very different. The former is an adrenalin state while the latter is not; they would need two different anchors, one for confidence and one for calmness. I often show the client how to set one in my consulting room and leave them to set the other at home. I usually suggest that the anchor could be clenching a fist, pressing a finger and thumb together or a visual image that they bring to mind. It needs to be something that they can reproduce exactly and that doesn't get triggered accidentally.

▶ Building a confidence anchor

If they feel that they have never felt confident then suggest that they ask their unconscious to come up with the memory of a time when some positive event happened. To allow their conscious mind to 'wonder' just what the unconscious part of their mind might come up with. To stop 'trying', but to just relax and allow their mind to drift with the idea of what feeling confident means to them. Maybe the first time they swam a width at the swimming pool or completed the obstacle race at school, maybe the very first time they baked a cake and it rose in the middle instead of sinking! What would it feel like to climb up a very steep hill and finally reach the top, where they can see the view spread out before them and feel the wind in their hair? How would it feel to win a race and have everyone cheering them on? Encourage them to use their imagination!

It doesn't have to be historically accurate – remember that it is the feeling of being in control and of being confident that you want them to tie into a trigger, so that anything they can do internally to increase the feelings will help. Make the colours brighter, bring out the sun, make it even better than they actually remember. Maybe surround the swimming pool with cheering onlookers as they swim their width! Encourage their imagination and above all, help them to ENJOY IT!

I usually suggest that the client do this with their eyes closed as it is normally easier to concentrate and visualise. I ask them to go back and re-experience the event they have chosen, seeing what they saw through their own eyes, hearing what they heard, smelling or tasting as they did then and feeling whatever they felt, whatever they were touching, whatever they were doing. As they do this, they can become aware of the good feelings they have and build them up and up, as they put in their anchor or link. It is important that they release the anchor at the peak of the emotion and not anchor its decay.

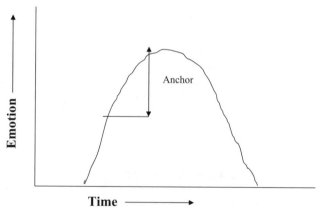

Figure 12.1   Setting an anchor

The anchor ties in the link between what they visualise and the good feeling it generates. Just as a muscle becomes stronger and more powerful with use, the more often they activate their anchor the stronger the link becomes and the easier it is to access it.

If they have a visual image that links them to good feelings, then suggest they keep looking up and imagining it. The more often they bring it to the 'front of their mind', the easier it will be to do when they are feeling anxious.

The client can continue to help strengthen their anchor by settling themselves down on other occasions and going back to the same or a different memory of a suitable time and linking the feelings to their anchor by clenching their fist, etc.

▶ Calmness anchors

I often ask a client on their first visit to close their eyes and tell me what kind of image comes to mind as I say the words 'Calm . . . peacefulness . . . tranquillity'. If they already have a good visual or auditory link to a calm feeling, then that can be utilised. If the client has developed special place imagery, then this will act as a visual image link to feelings of calmness each time they bring it to mind. Every time the client does their self-hypnosis and feels calm, they can activate their calmness anchor and build it up to be even stronger.

> Claire was a young woman who wanted to take her singing to a professional level. She came to see me with severe performance anxiety, which had led her to feeling nauseous and actually vomiting before going on stage. I taught her a confidence anchor and positive mental rehearsal (page 58) and she used pressing her right index finger and thumb together as her anchor. This worked very successfully and several years on, you can still see her activating her anchor as she walks on stage.

▶ Increasing effectiveness

It is useful to check with your client how strong the feelings are that they access when activating their anchor. To be effective, it really needs to score at least 8 out of 10 and if it is lower than this, I suggest my client do the following exercise. I suggest that the client stands up, closes their eyes and imagines in front of themselves someone who has the confidence or calmness that they are seeking. When they are ready, I ask them to imagine stepping into that person and actually feel that person's confidence or calmness. I ask them to activate their anchor and check how strong it feels. This nearly always increases the strength sufficiently. Sometimes just getting the client to imagine building the strength up as required will be effective. Some clients find that setting an anchor is more effective if they use the techniques described combined with playing some appropriate music at the same time.

▶ Panic attack controls

Using calmness anchors can be very useful in panic disorder. It is all very well being able to sit down and calm themselves by doing self–hypnosis, but clients need something that works instantly when they start with a panic attack in a supermarket. Some clients find visual image anchors to calmness work very well, others prefer the hand or finger clasp. I sometimes suggest that clients develop a colour of calmness that they imagine flowing down their body (maybe from 'Calm' written in the air above them) as they say the word 'Calm, calm, calm' in their minds, as the anxiety flows out into the floor.

These interventions need to be used before the full panic attack develops. Again, a time for detective work as to what actually happens when your client starts to get a panic attack. What is the very first thing that tells them a panic attack is happening? What thoughts go through their mind? What is the first thing they feel in their body? Once they recognise it, then they can use it as a message that they need to intervene.

One of the common fears that people experiencing panic attacks feel is that they are going to die or they feel embarrassed that they might pass out. No one yet died in a panic attack and reassurance here is the key. I also use perceptual positions in this situation to good effect. What would they feel as a bystander if someone else passed out in the supermarket while they were shopping? What would they think?

So developing calmness anchors is very useful. Sometimes clients have already done this spontaneously. When I asked two clients recently whether they already did something that helped them to feel calm, one reported imagining being surrounded by a blue aura and the other imagined being on the beach on holiday and hearing the sound of the sea. One client I saw imagined being under a waterfall that brought calmness and comfort, another imagined rainbows.

Singing a nursery rhyme in ones head also works well to stem panic. The words and the melody occupy two different parts of the brain (right and left) and leaves no room for panic.

> **A useful question – What do you do already that helps you to feel better?**

▶ Summary

- Anchors can evoke either positive or negative feelings – they act like 'hot buttons'.

- Anchors can be something seen, heard, smelt, tasted, visualised internally or felt such as the pressure made by pressing a finger and thumb together.

- To set an anchor associate with an event that evokes the desired feeling and activate the anchor – repeat a few times.

- The feelings evoked by firing the anchor need to be strong . . . if they feel less than 8 out of 10 then the anchor needs to be built up further.

- Anchors are most commonly used to help access confidence, in performance enhancement and sports performance. Calmness anchors are very useful in panic disorder and anxiety states generally.

- Panic attacks:

1. Interrupt the pattern

2. Use diaphragmatic breathing

3. Activate a pre-set calmness anchor

4. Imagine calm flowing down into the top of your head and the anxiety flowing out of your feet

5. Utilise the imagery of your special place to access calm feelings

6. Sing a nursery rhyme to themselves

CHAPTER THIRTEEN

Helping clients deal with anger

Although there is only one arousal state mediated in the main by adrenalin, the negative side of this can be viewed as three separate aspects with differing responses.

Surprise, where there is no threat and therefore no action is needed.

Fear, where there is a physical threat to survival or health and the threat needs addressing.

Anger, which arises as a consequence to a threat to one's emotional well-being, often one's self-image.

It is important to differentiate between these states in order to act appropriately.

Over the last few years, I seem to have an increasing number of clients come to me asking for help with their temper. This is often, although not always, young men being motivated to get help by a foreseeable breakdown in their relationship if they continue their current aggressive behaviour patterns. Alcohol makes the problem ten times worse.

Anger, of itself, is not necessarily bad. Feelings of anger may motivate us to deal with problem situations. It can alert us to the fact that an injustice is being done and can give us the energy we need to fight to right a wrong or take the action necessary in order to resolve conflict. Anger can be viewed as a cue to use our stress-coping skills, it can express tension and communicate negative feelings to others and it can give an illusion of control – but does not necessarily mean that we are resolving the problem.

But anger often disrupts our thoughts and behaviour and can lead us to say or do things we later regret. It may instigate aggression as we act out our emotions, and in some cases, may become a social role and give the person a social identity or reputation.

Sometimes we bottle up tension and negative feelings until we explode into a full-scale temper – but it is much better to learn ways to manage our feelings so that we do not need to explode! We all need to find some safety valves and helping clients explore and manage their feelings can be very rewarding.

Anger becomes a problem when it arises too easily and too often, is too intense, lasts too long or leads to aggression. It can take away our choices of behaviour if we allow it to do so.

▶ Suppressed anger

Sometimes anger that has been suppressed and unexpressed in the past can underlie a problem such as in the example below.

Ann – a Woman with Fibromyalgia

Ann was a 51-year-old woman who presented with a 'diagnosis' of fibromyalgia wanting help with her chronic pain. She had had fibromyalgia for the past two years, but a variety of non-specific symptoms over many years previously.

Her mother had died when Ann was 17 and she had married two years later. This marriage (to an alcoholic) had lasted 14 years and she had had two sons. When eventually she had divorced him 18 years previously, it had led to an estrangement from her younger son. This son was very angry with her for divorcing his father and took every opportunity to embarrass and humiliate her in public and within the family. He would not even allow her to see her grandchildren. Ann had remarried happily five years ago but then two years ago her eldest son had emigrated to Australia.

She had never felt able to express her hurt and upon my asking if she felt anger, she replied that she had been taught by her mother that it was not 'nice' to feel angry but maybe she was 'angry inside'.

Work over two or three months was directed at helping Ann express and resolve her feelings of anger and loss with a dramatic resolution of her physical problems.

▶ Causes of anger and arousal

Actual external events or situations may trigger feelings of anger but very often so do thoughts and perceptions about such events or situations. Feelings of anger and frustration may arise when someone is blocked or disappointed in an attempt to do things. Small annoyances or irritations, such as excessive noise or interruptions, stimulate anger when someone is already tense and stressed. Caffeine may also play a part and it is worth enquiring about your client's caffeine intake if they are having problems with irritability and anger.

▶ Find the pattern

The first fact we need to bring to our client's attention is that although external events and other people may encourage or trigger a feeling of anger, we actually make ourselves angry, even if we are not consciously aware of doing so. As this is the case, we can learn ways to help ourselves deal with the feeling more constructively.

As before – we need to find the pattern – and then it can be changed. The client needs to interrupt the pattern early on, before the anger builds up, or they will tend to get sucked into the emotion and it becomes much more difficult to interrupt it.

Anger is often a way people use to cover up feelings of helplessness, embarrassment, guilt or fear in front of others. Sometimes it is easier to build up anger and have a rant and a rave rather than face the underlying feeling of inadequacy. We may also feel angry when our pride is hurt, when we take criticism personally as an attack upon ourselves rather than on something that we have or haven't done.

I use stories from my own experience to convey the ideas I want to get across. For instance, I can remember how angry my parents were with me, when as a little girl, I got lost on the beach on a seaside family holiday. I was very happy sucking a lollipop sat with the Red-Cross lady. But I can understand *now* how my parents must have felt; worried and helpless, and feeling the implied criticism that they couldn't look after a small child properly without having her wander off! No wonder they were angry. Sometimes we can understand and resolve these feelings now, which may have been very confusing or frightening to us many years previously.

When we feel angry, we tend to focus on things that confirm our feelings of anger and this fuels these feelings further. As I mentioned before, we look at the world through the filter of whatever emotion we are experiencing at the time. We also build up our anger by going over and over in our mind the situation that triggered our anger and often talking about it to ourselves internally.

I think one of the reasons people seem to be having more problems with anger is their higher stress levels, so teaching anxiety management and self-hypnotic relaxation techniques can help here too. Remember too that someone who is anxious and stressed will lose their sense of proportion and their sense of humour.

> **You cannot be angry and relaxed at the same time.**
> **When you're uptight, little things seem like big things.**

We know that when clients bottle up their anger and do not express or deal with it, it may become destructive – both emotionally and physically. If anger is not serving a good purpose and the client understands whatever message the anger is providing, then it may be appropriate for the client to learn ways of letting it go. Suppressed anger can be very destructive, leading to many problems, not only irritability, impatience and raised blood pressure, but also many psychosomatic symptoms such as headaches, irritable bowel syndrome, skin conditions and muscular pains. Negative feelings, like anger, don't just go away if we put the lid on them. They stay around and influence how we feel and react to other people. Suppressed anger builds up so that one operates from a higher baseline of anger and is more likely to flare up and lose one's temper.

You could suggest that they write the person concerned a letter (but don't send it!) as an outlet for their emotions. By writing down how they feel it gives them some distance from their feelings so they become more manageable and less overwhelming. I have found this useful when it would be inappropriate for them to express their anger (maybe it would get them sacked, or maybe the anger is felt towards someone now dead).

▶ Silent abreaction

Another safe way of helping people deal with anger is 'Silent Abreaction'; using visualisation techniques to allow our minds to 'let go' and disperse these strong negative feelings. This can be used with a client during their consultation and then they can go and use the technique whenever they feel appropriate. Of course, you would have needed to have talked about self-hypnosis and the use of imagery beforehand.

In this technique, they sit down, close their eyes and visualise a place such as a quarry or a mountain, miles away from anywhere or anyone. There they find a rock that is suitable for their anger. They imagine projecting all the anger they wish to get rid of into the rock so that it becomes their anger, maybe marking it in some way. They can adapt it in any way they wish in order to link it to their particular situation. They then deal with that rock in any way that they think fit. It can be smashed up by a sledgehammer, a pickaxe or even a pneumatic drill. They can enjoy really giving it some welly! If they want to hurl verbal abuse at it in their head then they do so, no one will be disturbed. When they are satisfied with the end result and the rock is in tiny pieces, the anger has been dealt with. They then decide what seems right to do with the dust that is left and then allow themselves to imagine going to an appropriate place to feel calm again and bring some of that positive emotion back with them as they open their eyes and return to the here and now. It is very important to imagine a calm place, such as a mountain stream or a woodland glade, and to get in touch with those feelings of calmness first and not to open their eyes as soon as they have finished smashing up their rock.

An alternative way to let go of anger would be to suggest to your clients that they could imagine an activity such as bread making and work out their feelings as they knead the dough, maybe throwing the bread they have made to the ducks swimming on their imaginary river!

They could actually do this in reality so that as well as venting their anger safely, you get a tasty loaf of bread into the bargain! I quite often suggest this to young adults and children.

They could use Playdoh or salt dough to make a symbolic image and then do whatever work they want to on that image. Whenever they have vented their angry feelings like this, then make sure they take a little time to get in touch with calmer feelings before continuing with life.

In the 1970s, it was a popular idea to go and punch cushions to allow the anger expression! Young men may take up boxing or use a punchbag at home as a way of helping themselves release anger safely.

We can suggest that our clients who are having anger problems actually stop and think about what is happening when they start to feel irritated and then angry. They can start to be aware of various changes in their own body language such as averting their eyes, clenching their teeth and fists, crossing their arms, tensing various muscles, sweating, their stance, increasing restlessness, or maybe undertaking displacement activities (some physical activity such as cleaning or shuffling papers to try and distract from the feeling). They may become aware of internal thoughts such as 'You're gonna get it now'. As always, the first step is to become self-aware, to recognise the patterns and then to interrupt them.

We can suggest that our clients recognise their internal 'smoke alarm' for anger. One needs time to change internal emotions and behaviour. The earlier one recognises the signs the more time one has to create and evaluate alternative choices.

Similarly, it is useful to be aware and recognise the early signs of anger in others.

> **Recognise the patterns and then interrupt them.**

Suggest moving away from whoever or whatever is triggering the anger. This also gives a chance to evaluate rather than leap in with an unconsidered reaction. Going for a walk rather than escalating anger upon anger in a row often leads to improved communication when the two people concerned come together again. If someone is overwhelmed with feelings of anger, they are unable to listen and evaluate what is happening. Exercise allows the body to use up the adrenalin and then evaluation and communication stand a better chance!

> **You cannot react creatively or resourcefully when in the midst of anger.**

Suggest they could focus their attention on something else and as they distract their attention away from the anger-provoking situation they become more involved in whatever they are doing and begin to feel less angry. I well remember one occasion when my kitchen got the best clean it ever had – and the physical activity helped me to defuse my anger!

My grandmother always told us as children, to take a deep breath and count to 10, and that can work as well! It interrupts the pattern.

▶ Relaxation

You cannot be angry and relaxed. When clients become practised at self-hypnosis, you will find that they can often recognise when they start to feel tense and angry. They can then take a deep breath in, and as they breathe out, let the tension drain away. Using calmness anchors in this type of situation works as well.

> **Humour and anger are incompatible.**

If they can take a step away from the situation and see a funny side to it or if they can bring a thought into their mind that makes them smile, they will not feel so angry. Maybe suggest imagining the person annoying them as a cartoon character or change how they hear their voice internally to a high-pitched squeaking!

Beliefs that we have to have our own way, that the world must give us what we want, when we want it, are at the root of much of our anger.

An old zen saying I rather like is this:

> **Happiness is expecting the world, others and yourself to be as they are.**

Get clients to take note of their internal dialogue. If they can notice what they are saying to themselves as they start to feel angry they can intervene and change it. They can challenge or alter the things they are telling themselves. Instead of demanding something internally, suggest they try changing it to a preference, and it reduces the emotional temperature. This may seem contrived at first, as they change what they say to themselves consciously, but soon it will become almost automatic as their different thought patterns get established.

> **For example:**
>
> She must be home by eleven – change to – I would like her to be home by eleven.
>
> They have to tidy their room – change to – I would like them to tidy their room
>
> He should have told me – change to – I would prefer him to have told me.

Another habit most of us have is in describing situations, either to someone else or internally to ourselves, as 'awful', or 'terrible'. This immediately places it at the far end of a scale from 'Minor' to 'Major' and loads more bad feeling onto the event. Words that describe 'all or nothing' thinking also tend to increase our negative feelings (see Chapter 7 – Cognitive Distortions). Things are very rarely black or white but some shade of grey. Words like 'never' and 'always' fall into this category. Challenging this kind of thinking may be done internally, or out loud, and can start to change the feeling.

For instance:
'You never say thank you' becomes 'You hardly ever say thank you'.
'You are always late' becomes 'You are sometimes late, in fact quite often!'
This takes the feeling down a peg or two, to irritation rather than to anger.

▶ Perceptual positions

Teaching clients to metaphorically take a step backwards and mentally see the situation either from the other person's perspective or from that of an outsider not only helps them see alternative choices of behaviour but is a useful way of defusing anger-provoking situations.

> If you put yourself in other people's shoes
> you won't tread on their toes.

▶ Using imagery

Sometimes it can be useful to suggest use of imagery to initially defuse the situation. By venting the initial feeling of anger by using their imagination for example: spraying the perpetrator with paint, they can then perhaps take that metaphorical step backwards and maybe see why the other person is behaving in the way they are.

Remembering that anger is often used as a mask for helplessness, inadequacy or fear helps us to gain a different and maybe truer perspective. You cannot change someone else's behaviour but you can change the negative effect it has on you.

▶ Behaviour versus person

It is important, I think, to remind clients to separate the behaviour from the person. Just because someone has done something that they feel is wrong doesn't mean that that person is a totally evil, worthless person and never does anything praiseworthy.

Clients need to bear this in mind also when *they* are being criticised. Because they have done or not done something does not mean that they personally are worthless and a total failure – it just means they have done or not done something, that they have made a mistake. The easiest way to gain experience is by making mistakes; this is how most of us learn!

As with anxiety-provoking situations, you could suggest that they put the situation into a different time frame. What is supremely important now may fade into insignificance when put against the perspective of 10 years, a lifetime or centuries.

▶ Fuelling anger

I have already mentioned that the way we use to fuel and prolong anger is by re-running the negative experience that triggered the feelings over and over in our head and adding unhelpful internal comments. 'I'll beat the living daylights out of him when I catch him!' 'Why does she always pick on me, I hate her' '. . . off! You . . .' etc, etc.

There are various ways that you can suggest clients use to interrupt and stop the process.

They can take a mental 'time out' by internally shouting 'Stop' to themselves or imaging a red 'Stop' sign in their mind's eye and then imaging something that is linked to pleasanter feelings, such as a holiday, a favourite place or activity or a birthday treat. Some people who find they are frequently jumping into a thought cycle that leads to anger may like to keep an elastic band on their wrist and twang it to interrupt the cycle (see Chapter 11).

Suggesting that they physically move from wherever they are when they start on the anger merry-go-round can also help to interrupt it.

It is okay to have feelings of anger; it is what we do with those feelings that is important.

One of the problems with feeling angry is that we often vent our anger to the wrong person. Anyone around gets caught in the storm, whether it's their 'fault' or not.

If we help our clients work out any background anger (Silent Abreaction – see page 129) and show them ways to reduce their general stress levels (see Chapters 10 and 11) then they are less likely to feel anger anyway.

Aggression

Aggressive behaviour usually triggers one of two responses in the other person.

The other party may respond to attack by going on the offensive and the whole situation escalates as both parties dig themselves deeper and deeper into their entrenched positions. This may lead to one party acquiescing but with feelings of suppressed anger and a determination to win the next battle. Negotiation is unlikely and at least one person is the loser.

Alternatively, the other party may capitulate without a fight. If this happens, then we get what we want, but the other person will feel resentment and suppressed anger. This means we do not have an ally but someone who will hope that we fall flat on our face and will not take any spontaneous action to help us. We will deserve all that we get.

Dealing with other people's anger

Expressing their feelings

The first step is to allow the other person to express how they are feeling without interrupting or trying to make explanations. As we know, someone experiencing a lot of anger is not able to rationalise or look at things calmly, so trying to explain away the situation doesn't work.

Keeping calm

Remember strategies for keeping calm. Take a couple of deep breaths, let go tension on the out breath and don't take it as a personal attack. Remember also that their anger may be a mask for helplessness, embarrassment, guilt or fear. Allow yourself to look at what is happening from a different viewpoint, either from their shoes or from outside. Use your imagination if it helps. One bank clerk I knew used to imagine a bucket of water on a rope above her work station and if she had an abusive customer, she imagined pulling the string and seeing the angry customer before her all wet and bedraggled!

Break the pattern

The second step is to try and move away from the situation onto 'neutral ground'. Physically, walking with them into another room maybe 'where it's quieter', acts as a break state. The angry person moves away from the place where they felt angry and is then more able to act constructively. It breaks the pattern of behaviour. If it is not possible to actually move, then try and break state in some other way, maybe ask for their name and address or a contact telephone number. They have to break out of their 'anger pattern' in order to respond.

Acknowledge their feelings

The third step is to acknowledge to them that you can see that they are angry and upset. Do not join them in their anger but get them to realise that you have listened and understood how they are feeling. Sometimes it may be appropriate to acknowledge that you would feel angry in a similar situation or to direct their anger at 'the system' or some other third party that made 'the stupid rule'!

Negotiate

Take a moment or two to put yourself in their shoes and as well as helping you to feel more in control of the situation you may find that you can see some ways to resolve it. If it is appropriate, thank them for bringing the problem to your attention and maybe ask whether they have any possible solutions. Remember to use your rapport skills.

Apologise

If it is appropriate to do so, then why not apologise? Many complaints and conflicts would be avoided if someone had said 'sorry' at the outset. 'Sorry' doesn't necessarily mean that you are taking the blame, it can also mean that you sympathise with their feelings. Once someone has an apology or an acknowledgement of their feelings, they are much less likely to continue to fuel their anger further up the scale.

'I' not 'you'

Try out the effect of starting sentences with 'I' rather than 'You' in any potentially conflictual situations such as when an errant teenager comes home late. This may seem an unlikely way of defusing the situation but I recommend it.

'You are never home on time' is felt as an attack by the other person and so they immediately go on the defensive and attack in their turn. ('Attack is the best form of defence'). If however you say 'I feel very worried when you don't come home when you say you will' then the other person does not instinctively feel attacked and a rational negotiation is more likely to take place.

Anticipation and preparation

Sometimes we know beforehand that a situation is likely to lead to conflict and angry feelings either on our part or that of the other party. In these cases, it can be very useful to do a mental rehearsal of the situation. Settle yourself down comfortably, close your eyes and spend a few minutes doing self-hypnosis, relaxing or focusing on your breathing. Then imagine the situation and see yourself dealing with the situation, feeling and acting the way you would like to. Then imagine actually being that you and replay the situation as if you were really there, seeing and hearing what is happening and feeling calm and in control.

By using some of the strategies, I have described to interrupt the anger pattern and alter the way our clients think to themselves about things, their anger is less likely to build. They can still feel angry but maybe less intensely and as they notice *how* they generate those feelings in themselves, they can begin to take control of them.

> **Don't take life too seriously – you will never get out of it alive!**

▶ Summary

Anger – becomes a problem when too intense / prolonged / inappropriately directed / too easily aroused / leads to aggression.

We make our own feelings.

Anger can cover up embarrassment / fear / helplessness / guilt / hurt pride.

Anger can occur when we take criticism personally, rather than directed at our behaviour.

Recognise anger – notice the pattern – notice your own 'smoke alarm' – how do you fuel your anger – internal dialogue? – visualising event over and over again?

Recognise anger

Evaluate – am I in danger? – if so deal with that first – if not then *I'm angry*.
Intervene – to stop the anger getting out of control.

Focus of attention – Shift it away from things that don't matter or which can't be changed.
Expectations – If they are unrealistically high, you are going to be disappointed.
Appraisal – Separate behaviour from the whole person. Don't take things personally. Be flexible.

Anger interruption techniques

1. Interrupt the pattern of behaviour
   Time out – count to 10
   physical time out – walk away, close eyes
   Relaxation – breathing, muscular relaxation, imagery

2. Interrupt the thought cycle

       Self-talk – this can fuel anger or help prevent it
            – prefer/like rather than must/should
       Thought-stopping (a mental 'time out')
            – Imagery – stop sign, red light, 'STOP' or 'NO'
            – Nursery rhyme – occupies left and right brain
            – Elastic band on wrist – 'twang it' not 'damn it'

3. Defuse internal anger – especially suppressed anger
            – silent abreaction / writing letter /making bread and so on

Dealing with other people's anger / aggression

1. They are expressing their feelings – logical explanation doesn't work – so don't bother to argue!

2. Keep your calm – recognise that anger may be masking other emotional difficulties – maybe use imagery

3. Break the pattern – move position, ask for name/address, etc.

4. Acknowledge their feelings

5. Build rapport – remember representational systems, etc.

6. Negotiate – perceptual positions

7. Maybe apologise

8. Start sentences in a conflict situation with 'I' rather than 'You'

9. Anticipation and positive mental rehearsal

> **Don't try to resolve an issue when still feeling angry – wait for the adrenalin to subside – go for a walk first**

Useful phrases for constructive internal dialogue – use whatever fits the situation

What is it that I have to do?
Remember, I need to stick to the issues and not take it personally
I can manage the situation. I know how to control my anger
Now – don't take this too seriously . . .
As long as I keep my cool, I'm in control.
Keep focused on the issues, not the person.
I don't need to prove myself.

There is no point in getting angry – it won't change anything.
I'm not going to let this get to me.
It is a real shame that she has to act like this.
For someone to be that irritable, they must be awfully unhappy.
Let's try and work together on this, we may both have a point.
Hello adrenalin.
Getting upset won't help.
I'll let him make a fool of himself but I'll stay in control.
She'd probably like me to get angry. Well I'm going to disappoint her.
Don't take it personally.
Why not laugh about the situation, it's not really that important.
Forget it now and let's get on with more important and interesting things.
What a wally, how did he get the job?
I'll get better at this as I get more practice.

CHAPTER FOURTEEN

Helping build self-esteem

What do we mean by being assertive?

Being assertive means that we have enough self-confidence and self-esteem to calmly tell other people about our feelings and what we would like them to do. It is not being arrogant – which is a mask for underlying insecurity. If you are comfortable with yourself, then you are more likely to be aware and respectful of other people's feelings. If someone has low self-esteem, they often end up being a doormat, always allowing other people to determine what they should do.

Some clients think that loving themselves equates to being selfish. I would suggest that in order to love someone else, one has to accept and love oneself first, and this means taking care of one's own emotional well-being and taking some time for themselves. If your client feels that this is self-centred and selfish, they need to explore the motivation behind their selflessness. Usually, this is because they need to be seen as 'good' and need the external appreciation. Once a client has good self-esteem and is comfortable with themselves, they are freed from this driving force and can truly care and love another because they feel love and compassion for others.

If we do not feel and behave in an assertive manner, then we inevitably end up doing things we really don't want to do with an underlying feeling of resentment. We all have to do things that we would rather not do but if we have taken part in the negotiation and our feelings have been acknowledged, then we can usually do them with a good grace for the success of the end result. If someone has good self-esteem, they are more likely to be able to show love and care for others.

Assertiveness recognises the rights and feelings of others. Those who are assertive are also more likely to be happy. This is because they have a better chance of getting their needs met as they can communicate their feelings without being aggressive. Those who are aggressive don't get their needs met as often and spend a lot of time in needless conflict.

Many clients have emotional problems which poor self-esteem underpins, so in order to help our clients, we need to help them build up their self-esteem – to feel better about themselves – to ego-strengthen them. Many clients say they want to feel more self-confident. To be self-confident, the client needs to have reasonably good self-esteem and build a positive feedback loop with successful actions.

> **Self-esteem is 'being'**
> **Self-confidence is 'doing'**

So first we need to have reasonably good self-esteem. Some people need a lot of external reassurance that they are okay but all the reassurance in the world amounts to nothing if they don't feel that they are okay internally, if they feel worthless.

▶ How to build self-esteem

It is important to use any chance you can to boost your clients' self-esteem. Start by congratulating them on actually coming to see you. Often their acknowledgement that they have a problem that they need some help with is a huge first step forward towards where they want to go and it needs acknowledgement by the health professional to whom they have come for help.

▶ Mindfulness

An important factor in helping clients with self-esteem issues is encouraging them to be in the present moment without evaluation. Whatever emotional problem the client presents with, it is built up by having thoughts about feelings and behaviours. Then we have thoughts about those thoughts and so on. Before we know it, we have built an entire edifice upon a single thought or feeling. We need to encourage our clients to just *be* with a thought or feeling without evaluating or building on it. A thought is just a thought and a feeling is just a feeling . . .

I suggest that clients might like to imagine their thoughts as bubbles that just arise and then float away; they don't need to follow them.

▶ Dealing with inner criticism

Although we all have internal criticism to a greater or lesser extent, some people still manage to have a reasonably good portion of self-esteem! How do they do that?

We all have some form of negative internal dialogue, self-criticism or thought processing that can persist in telling us that we are a failure or that we did something wrong. This can be useful in that it can make us aware of where we need to make changes, but we need to remember that it is our behaviour that is being criticised not our person and if it doesn't seem like that, then we need to challenge that critical thought!

▶ Internal argument

One way that people deal with negative thoughts is to challenge them and think about what evidence there is to support the thought or not. They have an argument within themselves and the negative thoughts sometimes admit defeat!

▶ Positive parrot

Some people have a negative parrot (figuratively speaking) on one shoulder and need to develop a positive parrot on the other! They need to remember to say 'Well done' to themselves when something went well, as well as criticising themselves when it didn't. We are not very good in this country at praising ourselves. It is considered boastful. But anyone working with children knows that they respond to praise much better than to criticism and it is no different when we are grown up! So it seems only fair that if we criticise ourselves, that we also give ourselves acknowledgement and praise when it is due.

I well remember a client who described her critical voice as a green and yellow parrot sitting on her left shoulder. She developed a positive red parrot on her right shoulder that would give a positive and encouraging slant on her behaviour. She described this to her friend and her friend bought her a toy red parrot as a birthday present. She used to keep it on the top of her television to remind her to challenge her negative comments about herself.

Contradiction/challenge	Explore the evidence
But I often do things right!	What did I do wrong?

'It all went wrong – I'm a complete failure!'

I must remember to separate behaviour from identity	
I'm not a complete failure!	Was it all my fault?
I did 'x' well yesterday.	

▶ Changing the critical voice

You could suggest that your clients close their eyes and focus for a moment or two on where, in the space around them, do they hear their critical voice? Once they have an external representation of their internal dialogue, it becomes easier to change. Suggest changing its position and see if it feels better. If it does, then leave it there. Some people fade their internal criticisms into the background, or in some way, alter how it sounds to them. The internal criticism may not always be in their own voice, for instance, it could be in the voice of a parent or teacher. Suggest that they try changing the voice tone, so that it is high-pitched and squeaky, or a seductive burr, as this can alter the impact and emotional effect of the internal dialogue. Helium-ising the self-criticism is a favourite and makes the self-criticism less powerful.

▶ Distraction

Other people sometimes use distraction to negate the effect of negative internal criticism. They direct their attention elsewhere and ignore it.

▶ Writing it down

Sometimes it can help to suggest that if someone has a repetitive or compulsive thought, they write it down so that you can see exactly what they are saying to themselves. Then get them to change a word or two in it or to sing it to themselves in a silly voice. This often serves to disrupt it.

▶ Compassionate friend

Many clients with low self-esteem will admit to being supportive and compassionate if they have a friend in trouble. Unfortunately, they seldom activate this part of their psyche to help themselves and this exercise encourages them to do so effectively.

You ask the client to close their eyes and make an image that represents their self-criticism. They then listen to what it says about a particular event when they were self-critical and the feelings that that engenders are discussed. Usually, the self-critical voice is angry or disappointed and gives rise to feelings of hopelessness or of being a failure.

You then ask the client how they would react if a good friend of theirs was in trouble. The therapist then draws their attention to that caring, compassionate, supportive part of themselves that operates towards others in trouble but is rarely activated towards themselves. Having made an image that represents the caring compassionate friend 'part', they listen to what that part of themselves has to say about the event previously used to access the self-critical voice. The therapist then asks how that made them feel. Feelings of encouragement are commonly reported.

I often suggest that each evening the client sits down, closes their eyes and reviews a particular incident, preferably from that day as it will be fresh in their minds, and listen to what their compassionate friend has to say about it. We all know that encouragement gets better results than criticism and this exercise can be done regularly until it becomes established as an automatic way of thinking when something untoward occurs.

▶ Acceptance

Self-esteem depends on being accepting of yourself, warts and all. Allowing that there are parts of you that you would like to see change and grow, but that you have as much right to have joy of life as anyone or anything, else. We all need to give ourselves a hug at times, to tell ourselves that we are okay, it's just that sometimes we make mistakes and fall down; but we can get up and try again.

Sometimes clients need help to allow acceptance of themselves; their feelings from the past get in their way. If this is the case, then you may need to direct them to get some help from a psychotherapist or psychologist. Remind them that:

> **You are far more than the events that have happened to you.**

We exist as so much more than those experiences from our past, we each have potential, to be a loving, loveable human being, as much as any other human being.

Their parents may not always have encouraged and praised them as much as they would have liked or deserved, but as their adult self they can understand that their parents had problems and did the best they could. (Or if they didn't, maybe they also needed help but didn't realise it or were unable to get it.) So in some way, they could perhaps take that younger self on their knee and give him/her a hug and the encouragement he/she needed to grow that feeling of self-worth. With their adult experience and insight, they can help that younger self to grow a sense of being 'okay'.

Talking about these ideas with your clients and exploring what prevents them from being able to give themselves a hug can be extremely productive. Suggesting that each day they sit down quietly and metaphorically give that younger part of themselves a hug and the comfort that they need to grow can be very therapeutic. Remember that as you talk, your clients will almost certainly be doing internally what you are suggesting.

▶ Self-responsibility

Another facet of self-esteem is that we need to acknowledge to ourselves that we are responsible for our actions. We each sail our own boat on the waters of life and we cannot sail anyone else's. We may sail in flotilla or even rope up and throw each other fish, but we cannot sail someone else's boat and they cannot sail ours. This can be a frightening thought at first but also brings a sense of freedom. Many problems arise because people try to run other people's lives or fail to take responsibility for their own feelings and actions. 'You make me angry' is the obvious example here!

Increasingly in today's society, people seek to lay blame on others rather than admitting they made a mistake. The problem with this is that no one is allowed to make mistakes, the buck is passed; or they are so penalised that fear stops people from admitting them. But making mistakes is one way we learn!

Often clients may see us for help with their growing and often rebellious teenage children and some clients have great difficulty in allowing their children the space to grow and develop their own sense of self-responsibility. If someone is fulfilled through their children and defines themselves through parenthood alone, they will have great difficulty in accepting their children's increasing self-determination and independence.

The gardeners among us know it is important to prick out seedlings into seed trays or pots so that they have room to grow. If they are left with the parent plants, they grow weak and spindly, rather than strong and self-sufficient.

Encouraging such parents to develop their self-esteem by doing other things, beginning to branch out so that they have other interests as well as their children, is helpful. You often find in such cases that they have never done anything for themselves or their own enjoyment but are a 'martyr' to their families. Suggesting that they take some regular time for themselves is essential but often difficult for them to do without encouragement.

▶ Integrity

Integrity is vital to self-esteem. If we knowingly lie to ourselves or suppress and fail to acknowledge and recognise our true feelings, then we run into problems. As Shakespeare said 'To thine own self be true and it must follow, as the night the day, thou canst not then be false to any man' (Hamlet Act 1).

Acknowledging our feelings to ourselves helps us to express them more easily to others. If we don't express them, then people around us have to use a crystal ball and mind-read. They then often get it wrong!

▶ Go for it

We all need to have purpose in life, to feel that our existence is of some point. Not everyone has mighty goals, but everyone needs to have something to aim for, even if it is cooking the next family meal or weeding the garden!

Everyone, by virtue of their very existence, touches other people that they meet throughout their life and we never know how we have influenced things just by being in some place at some particular time, and not somewhere else. We are all threads in the tapestry of life and it is the links between the threads that hold the tapestry together. Knowing that you have a purpose, even if you cannot see the picture because you are a part of it, is another strand that weaves into our feelings of self-esteem.

▶ Good qualities?

One exercise I recommend to clients who feel that they have poor self-esteem is to ask them to write down a list of good qualities that they think they have. I asked someone this once and she told me she didn't think she could manage to think of any. She then brought me in a beautifully worked embroidery picture that she had created. We looked at the characteristics of someone who could have done this work – careful, conscientious, with artistic appreciation, neat, caring, etc. She realised that she actually did have these qualities but she hadn't thought of them as being part of her (see Case 2: Maureen). We all have some good qualities, so we need to get clients to acknowledge them and feel good about them.

Suggest they start their own fan club! Get them to write down at least a dozen good characteristics that they think they have. If they are having difficulty, then suggest that they enlist the help of their partner or friends!

▶ Pack of cards

One experiential metaphor I find useful here concerns a pack of cards. Take an old pack of cards (it doesn't matter if a few are missing) and ask the client to select a card that they think represents themselves, with Ace high and two the lowest card, ignoring the suit. You then take their card (in this example let's say a 4) and place it face down on the table. You then ask questions about their roles as parent, friend, etc. and get them to select cards for these, (in this example let's say a 10 and a Queen; and then how they think of themselves at various things they do such as gardening, sewing, cooking (say 10,

Jack, 9). These cards are added each time to the original card. You then pick up the cards, with the 4 showing, and confirm that this is how they see themselves. Then fan out the other cards and say 'What about all these then?' This of course can only be done when you know your client quite well and you know how to direct your questions appropriately so as to get higher numbers than the original card. Clients sometimes ask me if they can take their cards home to act as a reminder. One client finished working with me over several months and on her way out said 'When I first came to see you I was a four . . . now I am leaving a Queen!'.

▶ Self-image

The way we feel depends on the pictures we make in our mind's eye or the words we hear internally.

If we *see* ourselves as angry or lacking in confidence and *keep telling ourselves* that inside, then this will indeed be the way we will tend to behave.

If, on the other hand, we *see* ourselves as coping calmly and confidently and *tell ourselves* that we are feeling like that, then that is how we will begin to behave.

> **We cannot hold two opposing images and feelings in our mind at one time.**

Using their skills in self-hypnosis, our clients can regularly practise seeing themselves the way they want to be and, because they are in a relaxed state or in 'right-brain' mode as they do this, it will have a greater effect on how they feel and behave.

▶ Self-belief

We have all developed ideas and beliefs about ourselves as we grow and develop through childhood onwards. Sometimes it can be helpful to talk about this with our clients as sometimes they forget that beliefs are not set in stone but can be changed. I talk about how I used to believe in Father Christmas when I was a child but now believe that he is a historical or mythological figure, as an example of how we can change beliefs. I tell my clients that when they were first born they had no sense of self but that this developed over time. Their ideas and beliefs about themselves were generated by the words and responses of those people around them as they grew and developed. Maybe this would be a good time for them to review where their self-beliefs came from and decide whether such beliefs are still serving them well. If they have outlived their usefulness, then maybe the time has come to discard or update them. I usually suggest that they do this by floating up over their time road into the past (see pages 182 and 223) and as they look down on any relevant times in their past, to notice where and why they developed different ideas and beliefs about themselves. With their adult understanding, they can see how the people around them were operating from their own beliefs, emotional development and problems and decide whether to keep the particular belief or to consign it to wherever they keep old outdated beliefs such as Father Christmas. They can then replace the discarded belief with a more positive one that they think is more appropriate now.

▶ Saying 'no' assertively

One of the hardest things our clients (and often ourselves) find to do is to say 'No' to someone. We all sometimes say we will do something when our intuition tells us we should really be saying 'no'.

The first question we want to get our client to ask themselves is 'Do they really want to say "no"?'. If they are not sure, *then suggest they give themselves time to think about it.* Not everyone is good at making instant decisions. Taking time to think about it means that they can firm up their resolve to say 'no' and maybe come up with a kind way of conveying their refusal. Can they say 'no' with a smile?

If they really do want to say 'No', then remind them that it is worth a few moments of discomfort to avoid a much longer period of regret. Would not having to do something be worth the momentary discomfort of saying 'No'?

What would be the likely consequences of saying 'No'? How would we feel if the situation was reversed and they were saying 'No' to us?

> We often give other people less credit for tolerance than we would show ourselves in the same situation.

Get your client not only to acknowledge the other person's feelings but also to acknowledge their own and stick to their guns. Suggest that they avoid playing 'Persuade me' and that they don't start to rationalise their decision to the other party. If they say 'I can't do x, I am really busy for the next six months at least' they run the risk of receiving counter-rationalisations such as 'Then you could do it in six months time?'!!

> ### Useful Phrases
>
> I'll need to give that some thought.
> I'll get back to you on that.
> I really hope you won't feel bad about this but I shall have to say no.
> I feel bad about this but I have to say no.

▶ Criticism and praise

We need to teach our clients to separate the person from the behaviour. When we criticise a child for doing wrong we, let them know that we love them, but that we don't like what they were doing. But then we forget to do that for ourselves as we grow older. When someone criticises us, we take it to heart to identity level. Our clients forget that what is being criticised is something that they've done and that they are more than just the things that they've done. Too often, the person levelling the criticism is overstressed themselves or adopts a bullying role and gives criticism in a negative and aggressive way rather than sandwiched between praise.

So when our clients are criticised, they need to remind themselves that it is something that they've done that this person doesn't like or disagrees with, it's not they themselves. And the way we learn is by making mistakes, so maybe they can learn something constructive from the feedback?

And what about praise? When someone praises our client for something that they have done well, do they discount it or do they accept it? I ask my clients 'If someone gives you a beautiful present wrapped in beautiful paper with a big bow do you say "Oh, I don't want that" and throw it back in their face?' Of course they don't, so why do they discount praise? Suggesting that your client imagines praise as a gift helps them to accept it gracefully.

We should encourage our clients, when they have done something well, to acknowledge it to themselves, to give themselves a pat on the pack when it's appropriate. This is not boasting; boasting is blowing up what has been done out of proportion, but giving praise when it is deserved is one way of helping our clients do even better.

▶ Dealing with people assertively

It can sometimes be useful to coach our clients in what to do when someone is unkind to them. If we feel insulted, then we feel hurt and angry.

We then do one of three things. We can do nothing and just allow resentment and suppressed anger to smoulder away inside with negative consequences for ourselves and those around us.

We may go to someone else and elicit their support in our anger. The situation then escalates and bad feelings proliferate and spread. The atmosphere gets more and more tense and explosive. Of course, we also run the risk of further insult from them such as 'I don't see why it bothers you so much' or 'I don't want to get involved', which leaves us feeling even more isolated and upset.

Or we can confront the person who has upset us. Then the danger is that we may still be feeling angry and get further comments such as 'You always take things too seriously!' or 'I was only joking', which mean that you are the problem, not them, because you are too sensitive or have no sense of humour. Sometimes they may begin to explain how it 'really was' that we 'misunderstood the situation'. This does not usually help us to feel better! More often than not, the whole situation escalates and both parties end up angry, resolving nothing.

Anger needs to be acknowledged but cannot be resolved while both parties are feeling angry. Once things have settled, the client needs to be able to communicate how they felt, assertively but gently. Taking responsibility for their own feelings should mean that the other party does not feel attacked. 'Do you mind if I bring up something that I feel upset about?'

Hopefully, the other party will listen, thank them . . . 'I appreciate you telling me this . . .'. Acknowledge their feelings . . . 'I can see that you are upset . . .' and take some responsibility for the situation, 'I suppose I was a little sharp with you but I had a terrible headache this morning', which immediately lessens the feelings of anger and aggression.

Unfortunately, things may not quite go the way they would like, so the client may need you to coach them and tell them what they would like them to do: 'It would really help me if you could listen to me for a moment'. Then perhaps 'I feel "x" and it would be very helpful to me if you could do "y".'

The golden rule is to express feelings calmly before they become overwhelming. We need to coach our clients to express how they feel using the first person 'I am starting to feel upset' rather than 'You are making me upset'. The use of the first person demonstrates that they are accepting responsibility for their own feelings. It is important simply to state how *they* are feeling without apportioning blame. Then state what they would like the other person to do and how that would make them feel.

Unfortunately, in this less-than-perfect world – things may not proceed the way we would like and it may be impossible to change someone's attitude. Then it is a case of helping your client feel less threatened (maybe using imagery) and helping them to take a step back and see the situation from a different perspective.

One way of developing that different perspective that I find useful with someone having problems, for example with their boss at work, is to ask my client to tell me how they would view a bully in the play-ground from an adult perspective. What do they think he might be feeling; what do they think may be underpinning his behaviour? They can then start to see their boss as someone who might have personality problems and unmet emotional needs. They may even start to feel some sympathy and compassion for him.

Allowing ourselves to have needs, both physical and emotional, and acknowledging and fulfilling those needs, helps us to be more aware of other people's needs.

▶ The golden rule of assertiveness

The golden rule is to firstly acknowledge to themselves how they are feeling and then to let others know in a non-threatening manner before things escalate out of control.

I suggest that my clients use perceptual positions here to notice how they would feel in response to whatever they are intending to say. If it sounds threatening, then they could not only change how they say it, maybe alter the words, but also remember their voice tone and accompanying body language.

It can sometimes be useful to actually role play with your client how they would approach a particular person that they are having difficulties with and allow them to practise how it feels being assertive.

> **Express how we feel calmly,**
> 'I feel very upset when you don't let me know that you are going
>   to be late'
> then **state what we would like the other person to do**
> 'If you let me know that you may be late'
> and **how we would feel when that had happened**
> 'I won't then need to worry, and then I won't start feeling
>   cross'.

As our clients learn to let go of negative feelings, such as anger, they can react to things more constructively. As they build up their self-esteem and become more assertive, they find that they feel better in themselves, happier and with greater energy. They no longer need to behave aggressively and they can cope with other people's aggression more effectively.

▶ Summary

- Dealing with self-criticism:

    1. Change position and /or voice tone of internal dialogue.

    2. Challenge negative self-talk.

    3. Acknowledge accomplishments.

    4. Distract from or disregard negative self-talk.

    5. Write down persistent self-criticism.

    6. Develop a compassionate friend internal dialogue.

- Self-esteem depends upon:

    1. Self-acceptance

    2. Self-responsibility

    3. Integrity

    4. Goals and having a purpose

    5. Assertiveness

    6. Living in the present

- Self–image:

  1. Mirror exercise

  2. Playing cards

- Say 'No' when appropriate . . . with a smile.

- Accept praise and compliments as gifts.

- Accept criticism as useful feedback on something you've done – if inappropriate then acknowledge the other person has the problem.

- Express how you feel before becoming overwhelmed . . . own your own feelings.

- Let others know what response would be helpful to you . . . don't leave them to mind read . . . most people want to be helpful.

Examples of Positive and Negative Feedback Spirals

I'm alright	I'm worthless
Gives me a positive feeling	Gives me a negative feeling
I appreciate myself	I devalue myself
I form positive beliefs about myself	I form negative beliefs about myself
Increased confidence	No confidence
Feel I can trust others	Unable to trust others
I can ask and receive support	I can't ask and receive support
Happiness and increased confidence as I do more things successfully	Stop trying – why bother?
Believe that I have control over how I feel	Other people are better than me – may lead to inner resentment – may let others take advantage – may become a doormat
Actions lead to more success	Therefore I must be a bad person – self-destructive behaviours
Positive feedback spiral	Negative feedback spiral
I feel even better about myself	I feel even more of a failure

CHAPTER FIFTEEN

Helping with relationship problems

In any interaction between two people, 70–80% of the communication is at an unconscious level, mostly based on unconscious interpretation of our body language.

Our body language is determined by how we are feeling and what we are thinking at the time. It is amazing how a small change in one person's body language alters situations.

Memory is a dynamic process that involves reconstruction of processed information. We process information into visual, auditory, kinaesthetic, olfactory and gustatory components. Our response to this input is an associated emotion. If we change any of these components, then we can change our emotional response to the input or memory. Hence, if we can change the way we internally represent a person to ourselves, then we can change the way we feel about them. If we change the way we feel about someone, then we will change the unconscious body language, which *we* convey when we are in their presence. They will then respond in turn to that change.

▶ Bullying

A person's reaction to the client is triggered by what *the client* does, so if they want to change that person's reaction, they need to change what *they* do.

So if a client feels threatened by someone, then this will be expressed non-verbally in their body language. By using their imagination to see the threatening person differently, maybe in a pink tutu and Wellington boots, the client's feeling will change and therefore their body language and the ensuing interaction will change (see Exercise A).

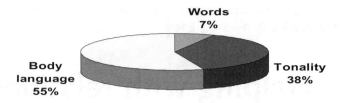

Albert Mehrabian (1971), Silent Witness, Belmont CA, Wadsworth, Page 75

Figure 15.1 Communication

By calibrating how they represent the person internally and comparing that to someone with whom they feel neutral, the client can notice the differences (see Exercise B). The client then alters their original representation accordingly. This doesn't mean that the client will like the person, only that the initial feeling the client has when encountering that person again is easier, so that the ensuing interaction becomes more constructive.

This sounds very simplistic but can have a marked effect. It works exceedingly well as a tool to help in a work situation if a client is feeling bullied. From feeling threatened and giving body language of a 'victim', the client can begin to feel more confident and in control, which alters the dynamics of the situation.

Practising either of these techniques several times in succession and then whenever necessary will mean that they will gradually replace the image that feels threatening automatically.

EXERCISE A

■ Close your eyes and allow yourself to relax.

■ Picture someone whom you find threatening and see them in a ridiculous costume or situation.

EXERCISE B

■ Close your eyes and allow yourself to relax.

■ Picture someone you have difficulty relating to and define *how* you see them: colour/black and white, size, position, photo/video, fuzzy/in focus, bright/dull, still/moving? (These are called sub-modalities.)

- Open your eyes and write down what you noticed.

- Think of something quite different, e.g. what did you have for breakfast? A 'break-state'.

- Close your eyes and allow yourself to relax again.

- Picture someone about whom you feel neutral and define *how* you see them: colour/black and white, size, position, photo/video, fuzzy/in focus, bright/dull, still/moving?

- Open your eyes and write down what you noticed this time.

- Think of something quite different, e.g. what did you have for breakfast? A 'break-state'.

- Look at your two lists and notice where there are differences.

- Close your eyes and allow yourself to relax again.

- Picture the person you have difficulty with.

- Change the relevant sub-modalities, one by one, of the person with whom you are having difficulty to the sub-modalities of the person you feel neutral towards.

- If the change improves how you feel then keep the change – otherwise put it back the way it was.

Remember that if you can help lead your client into changing their perception of the bully into someone that they could, maybe, even feel sympathy for, then the whole scenario will change.

▶ Relationships within the family

Young children react well to positive reinforcement and ignoring the undesired behaviour and reinforcing or rewarding the desired behaviour nearly always works.

When mothers come into surgery complaining that their children continually wet the bed, it often helps to get them to focus on the dry nights rather than the wet ones by suggesting that mother and child design a star chart; with stars for every night they stay dry, with a reward when they gain a certain number of stars.

Children need a certain amount of routine as this gives a feeling of security but they delight in pushing their parents in order to discover where the boundaries are. If parents focus on unimportant problems, then the important issues may get lost. This sometimes happens when parents become overstressed, so addressing your client's stress and anxiety will improve family relationships and allow them to communicate together better so as to show a consistent approach to their children. Sometimes it can be helpful to sit down with parents and identify what each of them feels are the important issues within the family. This could also be set as a homework task to bring in for discussion on a future visit.

Children who seek attention through tantrums and bad behaviour often settle if given some individual attention doing what *they* would like to do. Again, ignoring a temper tantrum is the best method but often difficult. Sometimes just holding the child until he or she calms down is possible. Using play to explore what happened can be instructional.

I love you but I don't like that behaviour!

Parents sometimes need to be reminded that they need to think before issuing a punishment. I well remember telling one of my own children that if they didn't behave they wouldn't go to the zoo as we'd planned. I realised, too late, that I really didn't want to carry out my threat as it would spoil the day for everyone else if we didn't go. If you issue an ultimatum, you have to carry it out or run the risk of being disbelieved and ignored the next time!

Another factor that needs to be remembered is that children under the age of seven or eight are not capable of abstract thinking. Delivering a punishment hours or days after the misbehaviour is not understood and the link with the misdemeanour not appreciated. If a punishment is used, it has to be done immediately.

It is also worth reminding clients who are using punishment or reprimanding their child to make sure that they separate the behaviour from the person. 'I love you very much but I really don't like what you are doing'.

With an older child, as with an adult, it is pointless to talk about what led up to the outburst until things have calmed again. Asking for their help and what would they suggest can be helpful. Often older children have very strong emotions but are unable to verbalise them or classify them, and suggesting that they take up some physical activity or beat the hell out of some breadmix or a punchbag can be cathartic.

If something isn't working – do something else! I find that writing a letter or a note to an older child often has more effect than continually asking or talking.

> **Positive reinforcement**
> **Give the child some individual attention**
> **Make a reward chart**
> **Suggest safe ways of expressing strong feeling, e.g. Punchbag**
> **Ask them what they would suggest you do**
> **Write a letter or a note to the child**

In a family situation there are usually regular patterns of family behaviour when tempers start to fray and the fur flies. If they can begin to notice the patterns that occur in their family then they can use their knowledge to interrupt the patterns and stop escalation. Maybe a teenage son is being wound up by his younger sister. All she wants to do is to provoke a reaction, which she then builds on, and so it spirals. If the teenage son suddenly turns to his taunting younger sister and gives her a round of applause, the pattern is well and truly interrupted!

If, when someone doesn't do something the client thinks they should, he raises his voice and shouts at them, and then they raise their voice etc, etc, then suggest he tries suddenly dropping his voice tone or smiling at them and saying 'It would really please me if you did x' and then leave the room. It may not work but it often does and rows get fewer and fewer.

If your client says that their children keep ignoring what they say when they are shouting, then suggest that they whisper or sing their request. Again, using less emotive language like 'prefer' or 'would like' instead of 'must' and asking rather than commanding will more often evoke the desired response.

Teenagers are often even more difficult and I often get parents coming in at their wits end hoping for some help with their teenage son or daughter. Here, I find that the most effective approach is to teach negotiation skills. The teenager wants to be treated like an adult while the parents still view them as a child. I suggest that the parents

"Do "X" right now!" ——————————————→ Child ignores command
Parent repeats command louder ——————→ Child ignores command
Parent shouts louder ————————→ Child shouts back
Parent looses temper and threatens punishment ——→ Child flounces out of room
                                                    slamming the door

Break the pattern! Do something different!

Figure 15.2 A typical pattern

prioritise their concerns and concentrate on the most important one or two and ignore the others for the time being.

> If we wish to be treated as adults then we have to behave as adults.
>
> The adult way to resolve difficulties is to negotiate.
>
> Each chooses the most important two or three things
> where they want to see change
> Then negotiate:
>
> If you come in by 10 pm on school days then I won't nag you about your homework.
>
> I won't insist on any particular bedtime and nag you to go to bed – you can choose, so long as you get up for school on time.

I suggest that both the teenager and the parents write down the two or three things that they would like the other party to do and two or three things that really upset them. They then bring their lists in to me and we spend 10 or 15 minutes negotiating between them. This can be done over several weeks with one change on each side each week. Patterns again need to be changed and rewards for change work just as well with teenagers as with younger children, especially when the reward is something that they have decided as suitable recompense together with their parents.

The sadder scenario is when teenagers go completely off the rails and refuse to work with you – they deny being unhappy with their current situation and blame everyone and everything else for their situation, refusing to take any responsibility for their actions. All I feel I can do in these cases is help the parents come to terms with the fact that their child has to lead their own life and make their own mistakes. The parents did the best they could within their own state of development and resources to bring up their children well, but once a child has grown older than eight or nine, the influence of parents starts to come to an end. All parents can do then is to stay in the background and be there for support if it is needed later. Unless you can build rapport with the teenager, you cannot work directly with them. Sometimes helping the parents stay calm and deal with their own feelings indirectly helps the situation at home so that things begin to improve spontaneously.

▶ Couples

This same kind of techniques applies when couples complain of continual rows and relationship problems. Encourage your client to notice the pattern of their rowing and then get them to creatively make a change.

If both partners are willing to work together, then there are various interventions they could try. One is to turn around as soon as an argument starts and argue back to back. This means that they don't get negative feedback from the other person and as around 70% of communication is body language, it is much harder to keep the argument going.

Another possibility is to prescribe arguments at particular times, in a particular room, each day. Each person has an uninterrupted five minutes in turn to say whatever they wish. This then becomes boring and the rows start to feel a chore.

Another intervention I have found very effective with some couples is to get them to replay their row in my consulting room using tonality or 'Ba, ba, ba' rather than words. This ends up in laughter and whenever they start rowing again, one hopes that the memory pops up and disrupts the proceedings!

Another useful ploy is to get your client to agree with their partner that whenever one of them starts to feel irritated or angry, they say a word, which has no emotional overtones, such as 'light bulb'. This then lets the other partner know that a row might be imminent. They agree whenever one of them uses the word they go into different rooms and wait for at least 10 minutes to allow feelings to calm down before discussing the problem.

> Back-to-back arguing – prevents negative non-verbal feedback
> Prescribed rows – time and place
> Use tonality instead of words
> An interrupt word

When couples have relationship difficulties, it nearly always comes down to communication problems.

Especially when there are young children, the partnership tends to suffer because all their time and energy are being given over to work and bringing up the children. Encouraging partners to have a regular time together away from children and home (where there are always jobs to be done or television to watch) each week or two, maybe going for a walk together or just going to the pub where they can chat about things, is often helpful. Time out has to be planned and taken – it is never just given!

Suggest that each partner writes down what they expect of their relationship, the things that they want and the things that upset or irritate them and bring the list in when they see you. Then spend a little time negotiating a change from both parties. It is the seemingly small things that make or break a relationship in the long run.

I sometimes suggest that each partner goes away and thinks about which behaviours within the partnership they would like to see continue and to come in and tell me the next week. This often spontaneously starts to help as their focus of attention shifts.

A game I sometimes suggest to try and change client's focus of attention from the negative behaviours is to ask each partner to break a pattern every day. Then each evening, the other partner has to see if they can tell which pattern was changed. People are more likely to have a go if it's fun!

> What do you expect from your partner?
> What would you like your partner to do?
> What irritates you within the relationship?
> What would you like to continue in the relationship?

A useful tool is the picture below that I have as an A4 sheet. If I have a couple come to see me that are always rowing, thinking that they are in the right and the other is wrong, I put the picture down on the floor between them. Of course from one side (partner A), it looks like an old woman. From the other side (partner B), it looks like a young girl. They make the experiential learning much more effectively than my merely telling them that they just perceive things differently.

▶ Summary

Communication – 7% words, 38% tonality and 55% body language

Bullying

1. Use imagery to make bully less threatening

2. Change sub-modalities

Relationship problems:

1. Discover the patterns and make a change

2. Write a letter

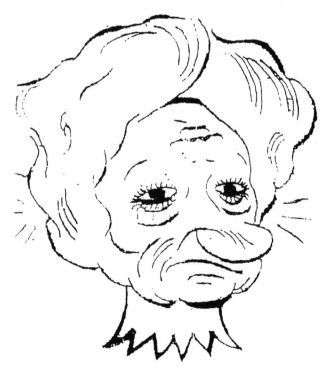

Figure 15.3 Picture – old woman. Turn page upside down to see a young girl.

3. Find safe ways of expressing and letting go strong negative feelings

4. Focus on the positive aspects

5. Negotiate

6. Use an interrupt word

CHAPTER SIXTEEN

Resolving trauma and guilt

Post-traumatic stress disorder

You may well have clients seeing you following traumatic incidents complaining of panic attacks, anxiety states, nightmares and flashbacks. Hyper-vigilance, feelings of heightened anxiety, feelings of needing to be alert all the time, are common following assaults and accidents. Often clients will have varying degrees of avoidance, from refusing to drive after a road accident to withdrawing completely from outside contact. Disordered sleep patterns are common and many such clients resort to medication to make their lives bearable. Nightmares are often troublesome; as also are flashbacks, the feeling that you are re-experiencing the event all over again with the sensory input of the time that may include olfactory, auditory, visual or kinaesthetic (physical feeling) modalities.

The DSM5 classification defines post-traumatic stress disorder (PTSD) as these symptoms occurring following a life-threatening event in which the client felt helpless. In my experience, they can often occur just as severely in the witnesses of such events or when the event has not been life-threatening but the client has perceived themselves as powerless.

Pre-morbid personality

Referral to someone used to dealing with PTSD is appropriate especially if the client has a poor pre-morbid personality. By pre-morbid personality, I mean how the client has experienced life prior to the traumatic event. If they have had problems with anxiety or depression, been in and out of many jobs and relationships, been on psychotropic medication, or had a traumatic childhood, they could be said to have had a poor pre-morbid personality and are likely to need prolonged psychotherapy. If, on the other hand, they had a reasonably happy childhood, are in a stable relationship, have had no previous mental health problems and holding down a job, then brief interventions may be all that is necessary.

▶ Flashbacks

In some the client with PTSD can be regarded as 'stuck' in a negative trance. In order to produce the flashbacks, the client needs to be at the higher end of the scale of hypnotisability as flashbacks are a 'regression' to the event triggered by some unconsciously noticed trigger such as a smell, seeing a colour that matched the car that hit them, etc. These are negative anchors and are as powerful as the positive anchors described in Chapter 12. Hypnotic or imagery techniques are therefore very successful in resolving such problems.

▶ Resolving traumatic memory

Any client with PTSD can be helped by simply teaching them some of the self-hypnotic techniques I have described earlier and by getting them to change the images (visual or auditory) in some way.

Often by giving the client space in which they can do this and by encouraging them to use their imagination to change their spontaneous imagery, the client can reduce or stop their flashbacks and begin to feel more in control. It is important that the change is one that the client generates and that the event is still recognisable. Any change begins to give the client the control that was lacking at the time and helps to redress the feelings of powerlessness and helplessness.

> John had been working as a taxi driver when a late-night fare had pulled a knife on him and demanded money. He came to see me complaining of flashbacks and anxiety. John decided that he would change the image of the knife to a banana. This also introduced a note of humour that was very therapeutic as he described himself being held at banana point!

> Steven had been in a car accident in which he had lost control and skidded headlong into a wall. He was suffering from frequent flashbacks and heightened anxiety when he came to see me for help. He described flashbacks of hitting the wall, which were mainly visual in content. I asked him to close his eyes and use his imagination to change the image in some way that would help. He suggested that he just see himself keeping control of the car and driving on home. After a little discussion, he realised that this was discounting the event rather than working with it and he decided that he would imagine the wall as sponge and his car as made of rubber.

In Steven's case above, he felt very angry and we needed to 'lower the level' before working directly on the event. I taught him silent abreaction as described in Chapter 13 to help him to let go some of his anger. This is a useful exercise to do before embarking on working on any trauma whenever the client expresses anger.

PTSD-type symptoms indicate that the client is 'stuck' in the event in some way. This is often the case when a client describes a past event as feeling 'as though it only happened yesterday'. These memories are always recalled very vividly.

One way of viewing this is that the client is stuck in a horror story without realising that the story had an ending. They are stuck at the point of being scared by the wicked witch without realising that the story ends with the witch being killed and them being rescued. One way that you can sometimes help is by getting the client to realise that their traumatic event had an ending. If you get the client to imagine the end point (e.g., being discharged from the Accident and Emergency department) and work backwards through arriving at the hospital, the accident and before the accident, it can sometimes be very helpful. Sometimes suggesting that they write the story of the event backwards can be used instead. If your client is very traumatised or has a poor pre-morbid personality, then this should not be attempted but a referral to suitable therapist made.

▶ Nightmares

In a similar manner, if someone is suffering from nightmares, suggesting that they close their eyes and imagine dreaming the dream with a better ending may often be helpful. They could also do this prior to sleep. Ensuring that they are feeling relaxed before going to sleep will also reduce the incidence of nightmares.

▶ Regression and abreaction

Unfortunately, whenever someone starts to describe some traumatic event, the tendency is for them to begin to access some of the negative feelings linked to the event and this is why, when taking a history, one has to be careful not to re-traumatise the individual. Too many people think that by getting a client to regress back to the trauma and express the linked emotion the trauma is resolved. Regression and abreaction may be cathartic but only when it is done in such a way that the client feels supported and connected to the present as they experience the affect.

One might say something along the lines of:

> And as you experience those painful feelings you can begin to look at me (bringing them into now) and *at the same time* know that that happened then and that you are not there, but here with me now. You survived and the older you from now can allow that younger you to be comforted and let go those feelings. You don't need to hold onto them anymore.

If spontaneous abreaction occurs then give support and help connect the client to the present while allowing them to express their feelings. Then direct them to experience something that can help them to access calmness.

Use of dissociated imagery – seeing and working with the event from a distance – is much kinder, both to the client and the therapist, and can be just as effective.

▶ Payback

Depending on the event, the client may feel a need for 'payback'. If someone has suffered an injustice or been harmed by another, they often feel a need to redress the balance. This can be done effectively by using the client's imagination, but it must be clear to the client that it is fantasy and not to be acted out in reality.

> Margaret had been bullied at school and as she pictured the event in her imagination, she squirted the bullies with spray paint.
>
> John had been humiliated and caned by his head teacher unjustly. As part of the resolution of this traumatic childhood incident, John imagined his head teacher being made to strip and apologise to him in front of the whole school.

The most important point about any traumatic event is that the client survived it. You might suggest that your client imagine their older self informing the younger self that had the trauma that however bad the time was, they survived, because they are from their future. This can be helpful in any negative event from the past and especially in road traffic accidents where the younger part 'stuck' in the accident has not realised that they survived, that they are okay.

(Interestingly this can be an underpinning of constant pain syndrome; the client 'needs' the pain to know they are still alive. In this situation, the client needs their unconscious to realise that they are alive and that they don't need the pain any longer.)

So, even without embarking on formal therapy to resolve a traumatic incident, there is much that can be done by using and changing imagery, utilising the story approach and teaching the client to take a different perspective and integrate what happened into the present.

Case Example – Sam

Sam was a nine-year-old boy who came into my surgery with his mother having suffered an attempted assault at the local park. He was refusing to go out and had become very clingy. His sleep was disturbed and he would not sleep on his own. He had already had his videotaped interview with the police and his mother was asking if anything could be done to help him. (Remember that if interviews, etc. have not already been completed or the case is likely to go to court, then one has to be careful that your interventions are not directed at the content as this could feasibly alter the client's perception of the 'facts'.)

Sam and I talked about how he was feeling, what he would like to do and what would have helped him at the time. I suggested that he might like to use his imagination to help himself. I asked him to imagine a television screen in the corner of my room and as he was a keen football player, I suggested that he might like to see himself on the screen playing football, maybe scoring all the goals. In this way, I was linking him to good feelings.

I then suggested that he could play a film of the incident in the park but as he watched it he might like to go in and help the little boy in the film. He decided that he would like to climb a tree and when the attacker came by he would pour a big tank of bright orange gunk or gloop over him. The police then came and locked the man away and Sam comforted the little boy and told him he was alright, that he didn't need to be frightened any more; just to be careful not to talk to or walk off with strangers. Then he and the little boy went and played football again.

This seemingly simple intervention made a significant difference to how Sam viewed his world and he rapidly returned to being a normal, happy nine-year-old and yet the consultation took all of 20 minutes.

▶ Guilt

Guilt is another negative feeling that clients often have difficulty with. One needs here to distinguish between appropriate and inappropriate guilt.

If guilty feelings are appropriate, then it is an indication that maybe an apology or some reparation is necessary. Appropriate guilt is a message that we have done something contrary to our internal code of ethics and that we have not listened to our 'internal voice' or 'conscience'; we have done something 'wrong'.

One of the commonest scenarios is that of a client who has caused the death or serious injury of another by their carelessness or lack of attention when driving. Here, the central question is what was the *intention* of the client? Were they intending to cause harm or merely exhibiting human frailty? I would also talk to them, as I would to someone who has been bereaved, that there are two fixed points in life; when we enter and when we leave. We cannot affect these, only the journey in between. This philosophy may not appeal to all but many people do believe it and no one can say that it is 'untrue', only unproven, as is any philosophical belief. They have probably driven less than perfectly on many occasions without such a terrible consequence. That that person's time to leave had come, does not excuse their carelessness, but may help them come to terms with it more easily. Some clients may find it helpful to regard themselves as 'the instrument of fate'.

There are various useful questions that can be explored with the client as appropriate. When will they know that they are ready to forgive themselves? What would they need to do in order to forgive themselves? If the person they injured or killed was able to talk to them, what would they want to happen? What positive element would they want to come out of the tragedy? These questions encourage the client into a different perceptual position, which can begin to shift them from being 'stuck' in their guilt. The client may feel that they need to make reparation in some way and the practicalities of this can be discussed. Suggesting that the client write a letter to the victim may be helpful. This obviously cannot be sent but can help the client express and begin to come to terms with their feelings.

There may be guilt surrounding, for instance, a termination of pregnancy that may or may not be appropriate and can often be seen as both. You need to be able to help your client take a step away from the situation and understand that whatever the decision was, it was made with her knowledge and resources *at the time*, and was what she felt was the right thing to do.

It is often the case that a vulnerable and insecure young girl gets pressurised by those around her to make a decision to have a termination and then forgets about this later in life when guilt feelings are resurrected by an event such as having difficulty conceiving. The client all too readily makes the belief 'I'm being punished' and feels that 'It is all my fault'.

Often guilt in these circumstances gets very muddled up with feelings of loss and sometimes it can be helpful to suggest that your client plants a tree or in some way mark their loss. Again the most useful questions to ask are what do they need to do in order to forgive themselves; and when will they be ready to do so?

If someone is from a Christian or Muslim background, I ask them what do they think about God or Allah – is he forgiving? Then how can they put themselves above this and not begin to forgive themselves?

How long are they intending to punish themselves? Are they actually punishing everyone around them as well? This latter point is often very relevant and often the client hasn't thought about it in these terms.

Much of the guilt, however, that troubles our clients, is inappropriate guilt and we can assist our clients in various ways to resolve these feelings.

Often a child will feel responsible in some way for their parents' relationship and behaviour. They may feel guilty about their parents' divorce or break-up of the relationship. This feeling may influence how they feel and behave in the present, especially in regards to their own relationships.

Inappropriate guilt needs to be re-evaluated; your job is to facilitate the process. Simply telling someone that they have inappropriate guilt feelings will have little or no effect. Again the way to help is to encourage a different perspective and using a story is much more powerful. I will talk about a scenario that is similar in some ways to my client's and ask my client whether the child in the story was responsible for what happened and whether the child should be punished for 'allowing' such a thing to occur?

You could suggest that they close their eyes and allow their present adult self to put their arms around their younger self that feels guilty. They can then give themselves some comfort and love. Their adult experience can help their younger self begin to understand that the guilt does not belong to them. This is something I find many clients can do and enjoy doing. In this case, and if they so wish, they can continue to do so on occasions by themselves when appropriate. If they have trouble then this needs to be explored further and referral to a qualified psychotherapist would be advisable.

▶ Summary

- Assess the client's pre-morbid personality
  Good = brief therapeutic interventions
  Poor = more prolonged psychotherapy

- Flashbacks – alter imagery in some way

- Anger – lower affect by using silent abreaction

- Imagine the conclusion of the event if appropriate

- Regression and abreaction should only be used if the client is fully supported and is at the same time connected to the present and their adult-coping self by the therapist.

- If spontaneous abreaction occurs, then give support and help connect the client to the present whilst allowing them to express their feelings. Then direct them to experience something that can help them to access calmness.

- Use imagery for payback if appropriate

- When dealing with guilt:

  1. Is the guilt appropriate or obviously inappropriate?

  2. If inappropriate, how would the client apportion blame if the same thing had happened to someone else? (i.e. from the observer position)

  3. Is there any message that the guilt is giving the client?

  4. When will the client start to forgive themselves?

  5. What needs to happen before the client forgives themselves?

  6. What was the client's intention?

  7. Is the client using the benefit of hindsight in their assessment of the event?

  8. Explore the meaning of compassion with the client

CHAPTER SEVENTEEN

Helping with grief

> You are alive until the moment you die.

▶ What is grief?

Grief has been described as a conflict between our feelings of what should be and what is. It can be seen as a complex set of physical and psychological reactions, which people experience following bereavement and which follow a similar pattern in most people (Hodgkinson, 1980).

It has been viewed as a 'state of mind' but more commonly is now described in terms of a process that the bereaved need to progress through. These so-called stages have been described in various ways but encompass accepting the reality of the loss and coming through the sorrow and pain of the bereavement to adjust to the change in circumstances, and eventually to be able to invest in new relationships.

The current approach to treating grief is to let it run its course and only intervene with behaviour modification, cognitive restructuring or working through a natural cycle of emotions when the grief process is prolonged, incapacitating or masked by a psychosomatic illness with which the client has come for treatment. The pain of grief is often not addressed and is in some ways a taboo subject as those around the bereaved are embarrassed by the display of strong emotion and feel powerless to help.

▶ Normal and abnormal grief

Grief is viewed as 'normal' or 'acute' when this process progresses over time but normality depends on the context, both cultural and otherwise, and there is an overlap between normal and abnormal grief reactions. Grief reactions have been labelled as abnormal if the bereaved has a feeling of well-being rather than loss, acquires symptoms that match those from the last illness of the deceased, develops psychosomatic disease, exhibits marked hostility to specific persons or shows a marked alteration in relationship to friends and relatives, feels numb and dissociated, acting out life rather than living it, or has a lasting loss of patterns of social relationships with general listlessness, exhibits behaviour detrimental to their own social and economic existence, e.g. unreasonable generosity or agitated depression (Lindemann, 1944).

Grief has also been viewed as abnormal if the grief reaction is of excessive duration, if the reaction is inhibited, suppressed or postponed or if it is exaggerated to the extent that the bereaved feels overwhelmed and resorts to maladaptive behaviour. Masked grief reactions occur when the bereaved seeks help for a physical or psychological problem unaware that unresolved grief is at the root of the problem.

▶ Harmless or harmful grief

I feel that grief is best classified or described on the basis of whether it requires treatment or in its relation to its effect on people – into harmless grief and harmful grief. Harmless grief is when it presents as sadness or sorrow, which even though profound, does not hurt the person, physically or emotionally. Grief becomes harmful when the bereaved person suffers hurt, both physically and emotionally. The hurt can start from the time of the loss or it may appear at any time after the death, sometimes days, weeks, months or even years later. Delayed harmful grief is usually triggered by some stressful or hurtful event. It may also be triggered by an event with similar emotional tags to those prominent during the time surrounding the last illness or death.

> Mary came to see me with overwhelming feelings of grief following the death of her pet dog. On taking a history, it became

apparent that Mary had never had a chance to grieve for her mother as she had to immediately take responsibility for the care of her father and disabled brother. When, a few years later, her father had died, she had been too busy with all the arrangements for the funeral, disposing of the house and contents and finding her brother sheltered accommodation to be able to grieve. When her dog died, all these feelings came to fore and led to a much more marked reaction that might have been expected. (See diagram on page 88.)

So how can you help someone cope with grief? I have found a few ways over the years that can help a little. Allowing clients to talk and to tell you all about it may take some time but is an essential first step. It is important to ascertain and respect any beliefs they might have regarding death and an after life.

▶ Two fixed points

I tell clients that I believe that life has two fixed points, when we enter it and when we leave it. We can affect the journey between but once 'our number is up' we have to move on. This, of course, is not everyone's belief but many find they can relate to it. So often we expect a client to die and they recover or, alternatively, someone dies when we least expect it. I also tell my clients my own views so that they may feel more comfortable telling me theirs. I tell them that I believe in some kind of spiritual existence after life, I can't prove it and if I'm wrong, I won't know anyway, but I think it is a more resourceful way to live one's life believing it! To begin with, you may feel awkward discussing spirituality but it can be very helpful and it is an important dimension of your client's experience that ought not to be neglected.

▶ Metaphorical treatment of grief (developed by Dr K. K. Aravind)

The wall of grief

Using metaphor can be very helpful in the treatment of grief. Grief is like a wall separating the bereaved from accessing the joy and value of their relationship with the deceased. The wall is glued together by unanswered questions that need answers before the wall can disappear. Encouraging the client to ask questions, whether it is about the cause of death, the context in which it happened or whether there was anything that could have been done by themselves or others to prevent it, is of paramount important.

The boats metaphor

Using another metaphor, it is as though we are born into a little boat, which sails on the sea of life. We each sail our own boat, no one else can sail ours and we cannot sail someone else's. We are carried across the sea of life every day and night of our life here. We cannot stop or alter the constant flow. We sail along during our life until we reach our final port, when we have to leave our boat and travel on in some other way. When someone we love dies and they reach their final port, it is as though we continue sailing along but have a part of ourselves still looking back and still connected to them at their final port. This feeling of being incomplete or of being torn is commonly found in grief and can only be resolved when we can finally accept and say 'goodbye' to the person we have lost.

Questions and answers

In order to do this the client needs answers to their questions. These may be practical as in the example below or may just be found through a discussion of what is 'is'.

There needs to be acknowledgement at an emotional as well as at an intellectual level that there are things we don't understand and have no obvious control over and that there are other things that we can control and change.

Often clients feel guilty that there was something they could have done which would have affected the outcome and this needs to be discussed and resolved.

Linda was having trouble coming to terms with her mother's death. Her mother had had ovarian cancer and had died in hospital. She had had a patient-controlled syringe driver of morphine, which Linda had pressed and pressed because she was so upset by her mother's pain. She was feeling very guilty and felt that she had caused her mother's death by administering too much morphine. I was able to tell her that the syringe driver

> would have had a maximum dose 'cut off' that would have meant that once the maximum dose had been administered, repeated pressings of the button would not have activated the driver.

Sometimes encouraging the client to take a different perceptual position by asking if it had happened to someone else would they think that person could or should have done anything different can be helpful.

Being unable to say goodbye or having had an argument with the deceased shortly before death are also problems that need to be resolved.

Sometimes writing a letter to the dead person can be cathartic. Getting the client to imagine what the deceased would say to them and vice versa can be very helpful.

> Seventy-year-old Greg was grieving at the sudden death of his son from a massive coronary. The last time they had spoken was in anger and although this had been a couple of days prior to the coronary, Greg was wondering if he had 'caused' the heart attack. We talked about risk factors of heart disease and that any elevation of his son's blood pressure during the argument would have settled long before the coronary happened.

Often it can be helpful to suggest that your client imagines meeting with their loved one in their special place (see page 111) and say together the things that needed to be said as they say goodbye. This they may want to do gradually over several days

Giving clients the space in which they can discuss their feelings such as guilt or anger, either relating to the deceased or towards 'fate' is really appreciated. Suggesting that someone does a silent abreaction (see page 129) can often be helpful if they tell you they feel angry.

Sometimes you may notice that your client has a focus entirely on the final illness and death of their loved one rather than focusing on the life that went before. Your aim should be to try and help them move away from the final illness and death, to which they need to say goodbye, to a realisation that they still have connection to all the rest.

One way of doing this is described in the following discussion.

The hands

You suggest to the client that on one hand (A), they imagine a symbolic representation of the deceased up to their final illness and death. They spend a little time putting there all the ups and downs of their relationship, the quarrels, the making up, the good times and the bad. On the other hand (B), they imagine a symbolic representation of the deceased's final illness and death. Your job is to facilitate the client in being able to say goodbye (B) so that they can receive the gift of treasure from the deceased to take with them (A) on the remainder of their life journey. What is stopping them from being able to say goodbye to (B) are the unanswered questions some of which have been described earlier. As the client asks the questions, the therapist needs to answer them until such time as there are no further questions. You then need to enquire what does the client need to hear from the deceased and what do they want to say to the deceased. This process may need facilitation or the client may just do it internally. Once love and forgiveness have been expressed as appropriate, the client is asked if they are ready to say goodbye to (B). As they do that, they allow that hand to fall and gather up the other to their chest where they can receive all that (A) means to them.

A further visualisation that I sometimes get clients to make when they have succeeded in saying goodbye is to ask them to imagine their future as a road in some direction in the space around them and to imagine all the value of the relationship that they had together symbolised by something such as a golden light or stars in their hand. I then ask them to scatter this out into their future and see it twinkling there waiting for them whenever they need it.

Someone who has been nursing a terminally ill relative may find that they have really done their grieving before the person dies. They may feel relief and often I find it helpful to actually suggest that they may be feeling relief or anger and that this is quite understandable – it doesn't mean that they loved the deceased any less. Clients are often relieved to have someone express what they are feeling and 'legitimise' it.

Sometimes suggesting that a terminally ill client write letters, e.g. to their grandchild, to be opened at various birthdays, etc., can be helpful in helping someone cope with the thought of their impending death.

Occasionally, a client has 'flashbacks' to some particularly vivid image, e.g. the person lying in their coffin. You then need to help your client take control of this image by changing it in some way. In this case, the client drew some beautiful velvet curtains across so that the coffin disappeared from view.

> Mary was troubled by vivid images of her dead mother with her eyes open and staring. She found that imagining that she leant over and gently closed her mother's eyes made it much easier to deal with.

You could suggest looking at old photograph albums and talking about the life of the deceased, this may bring tears but these can help in the healing process.

I am surprised at how many people find writing poetry at times of great emotional distress beneficial. Some already do this but others need encouragement to make a start.

As a health professional, you need to be alert for signs of unresolved grief – those minimal cues that someone is feeling distressed when talking about a death some while before. Unresolved grief can present in many ways, both physical and emotional, and being aware that someone has unresolved grief means that you perhaps need to give them some time to look at the issues involved and start helping them to come to terms with their loss. Often referral for grief counselling will be helpful if you don't feel able to help yourself.

▶ Summary

- Grief could be classified as harmless or harmful.

- Be alert to detect unresolved grief, which often underpins psychosomatic symptoms.

- Allow the client to talk and express their feelings in a supportive environment.

- Work to change imagery of any traumatic flashbacks.

- Work to change focus from final illness and death to the life of the deceased.

- Work so that the client can reconnect with the value of their relationship, which is always with them.

- Metaphorical treatment of grief

  1. Two fixed points

  2. The boats metaphor

  3. Questions and answers

  4. The hands process

CHAPTER EIGHTEEN

Psychosomatic problems

These techniques stem from the premise that we have mind/body links that we can activate to help ourselves. We all know that when we are very anxious or stressed any symptom is perceived as worse and is heightened as opposed to when we are feeling happy and calm when we can shrug things off more easily. But as well as helping ourselves to feel calmer, we can also directly influence our physical body by using our mind.

Psychoneuroimmunology is the study of how psychological processes interact with our nervous system and our immune system. It is well known that acute stress temporarily increases our immune functioning while chronic stress leads to a reduction in immune functioning and therefore predisposes us to illness.

The unconscious part of our mind 'runs' our body – adjusting our blood flow, our inflammatory response, our muscle tension and all our chemicals and hormones that influence how we feel physically. By taking time to sit down and do a self-hypnotic or relaxation technique, clients can reduce their levels of stress hormones and help themselves to feel calmer (See Chapter 11). Such techniques are often surprisingly effective in reducing pain or other symptoms that our clients may present with. It is often useful to ask the client to gauge the intensity and the 'bothersomeness' of a symptom as these are two very separate components. Only some clients will be able to affect the intensity of their symptom but most will be able to affect how 'bothersome' it is. If the symptom is only intermittent, then a measure of the frequency is also useful in order to monitor progress.

▶ Use of imagery

As I have suggested previously, using imagery and visualisation enables suggestion to be more powerful and more effective. You can suggest that the client construct or code a symptom in their mind's eye by focusing on the symptom and then seeing what image comes into their mind. It is important that the client is instructed not to have any preconceived ideas about this image; that they do not consciously 'try' to construct an image. Remember also that imagery may be visual or it could be sound or a feeling. Then they begin to change it in whatever way their intuition tells them so that it begins to become how 'it should be'. By doing this when in a focused, relaxed or right-brained state, it can often begin to affect the symptom.

For instance, a headache might be visualised as red and pulsating, which could gradually be changed to a gently waving blueness. One client with vulvodynia described her problem as a dark purple spiral moving very fast in an anticlockwise direction and decided that she needed to change its direction of spin and slow it down.

Once the client has an image, they can begin to change it for the better. Placing a hand on the tummy and focusing down to the gut can often be helpful for the cramps associated with irritable bowel syndrome. Work has been done on gut-directed imagery using the image of a smoothly flowing river. In this case, the client attends to the flow and adjusts it appropriately.

Although these methods can sometimes be effective, it must be said that often work needs to be done on the emotional distress or conflict underlying the problem symptom.

One visualisation I find helpful to teach my eczema clients is that of a 'magic pool' of the three Cs, coolness, calmness and comfort. They bathe in this pool and as they come out of the pool, a thin film of the three Cs remains on their skin to keep them cool, calm and comfortable until they visit their pool again. Alternatively some clients prefer the concept of using an ointment of the three Cs that they spread wherever it is needed.

You can also suggest ways of using visualisation to help in other ways, e.g. increasing immune functioning by imagining the white cells 'eating up' the germs in an infection or the cancer cells in a tumour. Many cancer clients find using their imagination in this way is helpful and it also gives them some feeling of control at a time when they feel that they have none. Some clients imagine that they have warriors fighting the cancer cells in their body; others may imagine walling off or starving the cancer in some way.

This same kind of imagery is often effective in the treatment of warts. I suggest to children consulting for treatment for warts and verrucas that they utilise the hypnoidal state as they fall asleep to visualise their wart being starved of oxygen and nutrition, getting smaller and smaller until it disappears.

Apthous mouth ulcers also respond well to this kind of approach and using client-generated imagery may be effective in cases resistant to standard treatment.

You could suggest that your client imagines a 'control centre' for immune function and set the controls for immune functioning where they feel intuitively it should be. They could have control centres for their inflammatory response and this can usefully be used in conditions such as eczema or arthritis. Control centre imagery can also be used successfully in patients with hyperventilation where they visualise 'their breathing control centre' and set it to 'normal'.

It is well documented that hypnotic techniques utilising imagery are useful at reducing the side effects of chemotherapy, such as anticipatory nausea. Professor Leslie Walker in Hull uses an olfactory anchor in such cases. He suggests that the client makes up a small pomander of suitable scents and whilst they are feeling well sniff at it 30 or 40 times a day. If they start to feel nauseous, they sniff the pomander and it acts as a positive anchor to feeling well.

You can also suggest they visualise a connection to 'healing' by imagining a colour or light flowing down their body bathing every cell and allowing them to be as healthy as is possible. This could also be imagined as a golden honey-like liquid that flows down the body bathing every cell as it does so. One of my cancer clients imagined her chemotherapy as a golden liquid that flowed around the black cancer shrinking it. Although our mind is the most powerful tool we have, it is too seldom used to maximise our body's health.

▶ Utilising unconscious resources

Another method of utilising unconscious resources to help with a problem is by setting the intention and using unconscious movement as a signal. We all gesticulate or nod our heads without consciously thinking about it and this method utilises this same kind of unconscious movement. This particular procedure is adapted from something similar that I learnt from Professor Harry Stanton and is based on the work on ideodynamic methods of healing done by Rossi and Cheek (Rossi E L, 1994).

1. Hold hands 4–5 inches apart and ask internally if your unconscious mind is prepared to work on 'x' now.

   If 'yes' then your hands will gradually come together as your unconscious mind reviews the problem and its antecedents.

   If 'no' then hands will move apart. Respect this and maybe try again later.

2. Allow one hand to drift down to your lap as your unconscious mind mobilises the resources it needs to deal with the problem.

3. Allow the other hand to move down to your lap as your unconscious mind starts to use these resources to help you with the problem.

It is important with this not to make your hands move or stop them moving but to let them please themselves.

This method is particularly effective for headaches and migraine if used early enough and I have taught it to many of my clients. However, it could be used to self-help with any problem or difficulty as it is non-specific until you set the intention.

▶ Causes of psychosomatic symptoms

If you believe the premise that all symptoms or behaviour have a positive intention, that they were generated at the time to help the person cope in some way, then treatment of psychosomatic illness should involve finding alternative ways of satisfying the need previously served by the symptom. This is most easily done in the hypnotic state as often this is not something accessible to the conscious mind. If it could have been done consciously, then the client would most probably have already resolved the problem. Although the health professional working with a client in this way would need training in hypnotic techniques, there are some simple questions and processes that may be useful without any formal hypnotic induction.

▶ Conflict

Sometimes symptoms arise because we know we ought to do one thing but we want to do the opposite or when there is indecision regarding two courses of action. You can suggest that the client closes their eyes and consider this, and then maybe use the Stanton's Hands procedure described above.

Shall I change from job 'x' to job 'y'?

Advantages	Importance (out of 10)	Disadvantages	Importance (out of 10)
Nearer home	8	Less pay	8
Starts later	5	Later home in evening	6
Interesting	9	Won't know people	5
etc		etc	
Total score		Total score	

Question	Answers	Score ?/10 importance	Question	Answers	Score ?/10 importance
What positive things might happen if I take job 'y'?			What negative things might happen if I do take job 'y'?		
What positive things might happen if I don't take job 'y'?			What negative things might happen if I don't take job 'y'?		

Figure 18.1   Example of decision grids

I have sometimes taught clients the use of a decision grid when they are undecided between courses of action.

▶ Organ language

If you listen carefully to what your clients say, anatomical metaphors abound: 'I feel as if I am being stabbed in the back', 'He gets under my skin' or 'It's a pain in the neck'.

You can suggest that the client closes their eyes and consider that, by using symptom 'X', is their unconscious mind trying to tell them something?

Once the connection has been made and acknowledged, an alternative may be found if needed. Alternatively, you could continue to explore the client-generated imagery . . . 'What do you need to do to take the knife out?' . . . 'What do you experience as he gets under your skin? What is happening? What do you need to do for it to feel better?' . . . 'How could you help your neck to feel more comfortable?'

▶ Serving a purpose – secondary gain

This needs approaching sensitively and often the positive gain of the symptom is not recognised consciously but it may be that the symptom appears to solve a problem. I tell clients how I always used to contract a bad viral illness early in January, which necessitated a couple of days spent in bed. Eventually I realised that it was a way of having some time out after all the frenetic family activity around Christmas and New Year. Once I realised this, I was able to ensure that I did something to reduce my stress levels at that time and have not had a viral illness in January since.

You can suggest that the client closes their eyes and consider that, although they do not want symptom X, is there at least one aspect of their life that benefits because they have symptom X? They can then start to find alternative solutions that do not require the secondary gain symptom.

Past traumatic experience

This could be an emotionally charged event, which gave rise to immediate symptoms or which served as a sensitising event that was activated by later events.

You can suggest that the client closes their eyes and consider this premise and then use imagery as described in Chapter 16 on the resolution of trauma.

Identification

This occurs when the client has an empathic relationship with someone, who is often deceased. As a GP, I often had clients who complained of symptoms similar to a relative who had just died; headaches following someone dying with a brain tumour; stomach ache following a death with colon cancer and so on.

You can suggest that the client closes their eyes and consider the question of whether there was someone close to them who had symptom X or similar? Once the link is acknowledged and any negative feelings of anger or loss associated with that person resolved, then the symptom usually disappears.

Self-punishment

We should be alert for this whenever we hear, 'If only'. This may occur with appropriate and inappropriate guilt (see Chapter 16).

You can suggest that the client closes their eyes and consider whether symptom X is some sort of punishment? One then needs to work towards resolution, often self-forgiveness, 'What needs to happen so that you can begin to forgive yourself?'

You could use a 'Compassionate Mind' approach: 'Whatever they did, they did within the context of what happened and their resources at the time . . .'. Looking back with hindsight we often forget how it actually was when we made a decision. A useful question might be 'Did they intend harm at the time?'

It is often useful to work with the client's spirituality . . . Is their God a forgiving God? If so, then would their God forgive them? 'Are you then saying that your standards are greater than your God's?'

▶ Imprint

This occurs when something is said when the client is in a vulnerable state, maybe as a child or in states of high anxiety or shock, that is accepted virtually unchallenged and becomes a belief throughout the rest of their life unless addressed.

You can suggest that the client closes their eyes and consider whether symptom X relates to something that someone has said to them. Once they have become aware of the connection and resolved the feelings around it, the symptom resolves.

In all these cases, it is important that the client rests in the question rather than tries to find an answer. If you have no counselling or psychotherapy training, then it is probably better not to explore psychosomatic symptoms formally and just help clients with using imagery. But if you are aware of these causes, you may find that you can help your client more effectively by picking up and expanding on something that they come up with spontaneously.

▶ Pre-state anchors

We have talked about negative and positive anchors and this is a method used to anchor a time before the problem arose.

You suggest that the client close their eyes and go back in their imagination and experience a time before the problem and set an anchor to this time. This is usually a hand clasp and they then squeeze their hand whenever they need to.

▶ Asthma

This is especially useful for helping asthma when the client anchors a time when they were breathing easily or before they had asthma, which they access as soon as they start to feel tight. With an asthmatic, do remember to tell the client to check their peak flow rates. It can be dangerous if, when you teach an asthmatic self-hypnosis for relaxation, they stop their inhalers because they feel so calm and relaxed; because adrenalin is a very effective bronchodilator. You need to get the client to change their physiology by using imagery to reduce the inflammatory response in their lungs as well as to open up their airways. Peak flows must be checked before medication is reduced or stopped.

Pre-state anchors can also be used for conditions such as migraine, eczema and psoriasis.

Firing a calmness anchor can sometimes abort an epileptic attack if used in the prodromal stage.

▶ Nocturnal enuresis

I often have mothers come with their children complaining of nocturnal enuresis, and with young children, I suggest that mother and child draw pictures to this story:

I would like to tell you a story about Mr Bladder and Mr. Brain

Mr Bladder lives near the bottom of your tummy and stores any water that your body doesn't need. At the bottom of Mr Bladder is a little tap that opens to let you wee and shuts when you are busy playing and don't want to wee.

Now Mr Brain lives in your head and did you know that your Mr Brain is a bit like a magic computer? It does lots of things – like move your legs when you walk and help you find the right words when you want to talk. It also tells the tap at the bottom of Mr Bladder when to open and when to stay shut. He is very clever!

Sometimes when you are deeply asleep Mr Brain goes to sleep too and doesn't hear Mr Bladder telling him when you need to wee. Mr Bladder tries and shouts but if he is full, he just has to wee!

So what I would like you to do every night, when you snuggle down in your bed, just before you go to sleep, is to speak to Mr Brain and ask him to keep just a little bit awake so that if Mr Bladder sends him a message he can hear it and wake you up to go for a wee. Maybe if he needs to go to sleep, you could ask Mr Brain to tell Mr Bladder to keep his tap tight shut until Mr Brain wakes up again.

You can help Mr Brain and Mr Bladder to talk to each other and then they can both say 'Thank you' and you can have a good sleep and wake up all comfortable in the morning!

Accompanied by a reward chart this often does the trick.

With an older child suggesting that each night just as they fall asleep (when in that drowsy, daydreamy state) they think about this story or a more grown up version of it often helps. Also helpful can be a positive mental rehearsal of the child waking up when appropriate, going to the toilet and then back to bed.

▶ Pain

Although pain is not usually regarded as psychosomatic, there is a large emotional component to any pain. Acute pain is often accompanied by high levels of anxiety or shock, which means that the person is in an altered state spontaneously. This can be utilised to give direct suggestions of comfort and coolness in the case of burns. People have a remarkable ability under these conditions to slow down bleeding and turn off pain if they are asked to do so. They may not know consciously how to do it but they can ask and trust their unconscious to do it for them.

One summer we were staying with friends and had a barbecue in their terraced garden. Their little boy, who was six at the time, came running down the steps at the side of the barbecue grill and stumbled. He steadied himself by putting his hand on the red-hot grill. While carrying him into the kitchen and placing his burnt hand under the cold tap, I continually talked about how he had been playing with snow the previous Christmas and did he remember how cold the snow had made his hands when he had been making snowballs. Within a few moments, he was engaging with the implied suggestions and his burn healed very rapidly with no blistering or scar.

In chronic pain, there is often associated depression and the client feels out of control. Again measures of intensity and bothersomeness are useful and client-generated metaphor and imagery can be very effective. Finding out when and where the client feels most comfortable and directing their attention towards this can be helpful. Self-hypnotic techniques are often effective in reducing pain and can give the client back a measure of control. A useful suggestion to use is: When everything that can be done and should be done has been done, there is no longer any reason to have the pain (Kane S, 2004).

▶ Negative suggestion

Remember that when a health professional speaks to a client, they are usually perceived to be an authority figure. Any utterances may have a greater effect than you realise, especially if the client is anxious or in shock. If this was always used in a positive manner, there would be no problem but the difficulty lies with having to have 'informed consent' for any procedure or treatment. This all too often means that side effects and possible negative outcomes are focused upon and negative suggestion is then given when the client is in a vulnerable position.

While in a state of anxiety or shock, the client will be processing in a more 'right brained' manner and will thus be reacting emotionally rather than in an intellectual and abstract way. Because people in shock, or when highly anxious, are in an altered state, imprints are more likely to occur and unwise remarks can have long-lasting and unforeseen consequences. It is important that health professionals are aware of this and take care both when attending accidents, in accident and emergency departments and when in operating theatres. Negative comments should be avoided and anything said should be couched in positive terms.

'You're finished' . . . may be interpreted at an unconscious level as 'I am going to die' and give rise to increased morbidity. Why not say 'We've completed the procedure and you're doing really well'?

So in these days of litigation, how can we convey to our clients what we are required to without focusing on the negative?

Instead of just giving statistics, relate it to something that the client understands and put it in perspective. As an example: ask your client how many people have showers at home with a warning posted, 'This floor may be slippery when wet?' Of course, the client will reply

'None'. But some people do slip over and injure themselves in the shower. Most hotels have a notice posted in the bathrooms but that does not mean that it is more likely that you will slip. As health professionals, we have to act like the hotel and give the warning but the actual incidence of someone 'slipping' may be very low.

Ensure that you leave your client with a positive suggestion such as 'Although we have been talking about some possibilities, there are always many possibilities such as a tornado sweeping through this hospital tomorrow. But it is not very probable'. You don't need to spell out the analogy; the client will take the point. Endeavour then to refer to an event in the future that the client has talked about, which will imply that the client will survive to take part in the event. 'When you go and visit your granddaughter next month . . .'.

There are certain words that the health professional should aim to avoid, such as jab and pain. Why not talk about a vaccination, or in obstetrics why not talk about contractions or feelings of pressure? Find ways of using words such as comfortable instead. Instead of saying 'You can use the PCA (patient controlled analgesia) machine whenever you have pain' why not try saying 'You might be surprised at how comfortable you feel after the procedure (try not to use the words operation or surgery that tend to have negative connotations); and in order to feel even more comfortable, you can use the PCA machine whenever you feel it necessary.'

Most good anaesthetists already give positive suggestion to their clients but this practice needs to be much more widely utilised. As the client is entering anaesthesia, they are in a much more receptive state than when fully 'conscious' and suggestions that they will soon be feeling much better, healing well and quickly have been shown to have an effect on post-operative morbidity (Lebovits *et al.*, 1999, Montgomery *et al.*, 2002).

Giving suggestions that the client will soon feel hungry and enjoy eating or drinking will often work more effectively to counteract postoperative nausea and vomiting than a more direct approach. One should also be aware of the implied suggestion of having a vomit bowl handy if someone is undergoing chemotherapy. Why not suggest that the water and bowl is there 'In case they wish to rinse their mouth out'.

Remember that how you present a medication or treatment will have an effect on how successful it is. The efficacy of a medication will be much less if the health professional says something like: 'Well, we'll try these ones. If you're not feeling better in a week or two we'll need to change them and try something else. If you get side effects then try and continue taking them for a couple of days in case they subside' than if they say something like: 'I would like to try you on these tablets ... they are very effective and if you did get any side effects they will almost certainly disappear within a day or two'. If the client has problems, you can be sure they will be back without you suggesting it!

▶ **Summary**

- Monitor symptom with scales of intensity, bothersomeness and frequency

- Use client-generated imagery

    1. Client focuses on symptom

    2. Allows imagery to develop

    3. Makes a helpful change

- Use constructed images

    1. Flowing river for IBS

    2. Magic pool or ointment for eczema or psoriasis

    3. White cells 'eating up' or attacking germs or cancer cells

    4. Warts or verrucas being 'starved' and shrinking

    5. Imaging the desired end result, e.g. pale smooth skin in cases of eczema

    6. Control centre imagery – immune function, inflammatory response, breathing, pain

    7. Connection to 'healing'

- Anchors

    1. Olfactory anchor for helping with side effects of chemotherapy

    2. Pre-state anchor in conditions such as asthma and migraine

    3. Calmness anchor

- Pain

    1. Acute pain – associated with anxiety or shock – give direct simple suggestion

2. Chronic pain – often associated with depression – may need exploration

3. Use client-generated imagery

4. Imagery of control centres, dials etc

- Avoid negative suggestion

  1. Avoid using certain words such as jab, pain etc

  2. Give information in a way that the client can relate to

  3. Ensure that a negative possibility is not viewed by the client as the most probable

  4. Give a positive perspective, don't leave the negative as the last thing the client remembers

  5. Connect the client to a positive future prospect

CHAPTER NINETEEN

Conclusion

This book has been, hopefully, a practical run through various ways a health professional can assist and help a patient presenting with emotional distress. It is not rocket science, but like most effective things, quite simple. It depends more on a change in mindset of the health professional than any deep and profound knowledge. It takes many things that you probably already know and places them in a context that enables our brains to process and make change.

As with any new skill, as our clients begin to put these strategies into practice, they will be consciously aware of what they are doing and it may feel a little strange. If they stick with it, then gradually it will become an established pattern that appears to arise spontaneously.

Remind them of the time when they learnt to swim or drive a car. To begin with, it felt difficult and awkward. As they became more practised, they started to do it without consciously thinking about it. It became a new established pattern of habitual thinking and behaviour.

The Four Stages of Learning

Unconscious incompetence
  – you don't know that you don't know

Conscious incompetence
  – you know you don't know as you start to learn

Conscious competence
  – you have learnt how to do it but it takes concentration

Unconscious competence
  – you do it automatically (or without thinking about it)

The most important message is first gain rapport! Without rapport, you will not communicate effectively.

Seed ideas with your patients at every chance you get – it is your job to help them form new perspectives.

Take a history – many solutions are more obvious if you know where the person is coming from – but ask for the Readers Digest version!

Find out *how* rather than *why* your patient is distressed, but remember to balance validation of their emotional state with a solution focus.

Become sensitive to and aware of your client's non-verbal communications. Use your eyes, ears, and your intuition, and do not take note only of the words your client is using.

Notice the words as well and use them for change.

Your patient will often tell you what they really need – if you have the acuity to notice.

If your patient can really connect with the way they want to be then they are half way there – at least!

Principles of Suggestion

Repetition increases effectiveness
Vividness increases effectiveness
Strong emotion increases effectiveness
Positive phrasing increases effectiveness
If you think you can't – trying won't succeed!
Don't judge your neighbour until you've walked a mile in his
 shoes
Worry is interest paid on something that may never happen
When you bury the hatchet, don't mark the spot
Use the past as a springboard, not as a settee
Happiness is contagious – be a carrier
May your God go with you!

Client handout

- **How** do you do anxiety?

- What do you do differently when you are not feeling stressed?

- Be very specific – what behaviour are you doing, what pictures are you seeing in your mind's eye, what are you telling yourself / thinking about?

- Smoke alarm – what is the very first thing you notice when you start to feel anxious or stressed?

- Do something different **then** to break the pattern, before the fire takes hold.

- Breathing Exercise (1) – place hands below lower ribs – imagine air flowing in and out through your fingers – starts to use the diaphragm

- Breathing Exercise (2) – close eyes and watch your breathing – the rise and fall of your chest – follow the breath in and out – don't try to change anything – just be with your breathing –then focus your attention down to the difference in temperature in the air you breathe out which is slightly warmer than the air you breathe in – after a few minutes focus on that split second when your in-breath becomes your out-breath, and your out-breath becomes your in-breath . . . maybe then visualise a patch of blue sky with a great bird flying – the wings beating in time with your breathing or take yourself in imagination to a calm, relaxing place.

- Body scan – check regularly whether you are holding muscles tight—let go consciously on the out-breath

© Ann Williamson 2008

- Mindfullness exercises – connect with the present – become aware of what you are seeing, hearing, smelling but without judgment or comment

- Body language – stand up straight and look up to feel more confident – if you are feeling low go for a walk and notice the chimney tops

- Revivification – or re-experiencing a time when you felt confident, in control, happy, exhilarated etc – use all the senses and then

- Anchor – ties in the link between what you visualise and the good feeling it generates to a clenched fist or pressing together of a finger and thumb – the more often you bring it to the 'front of your mind' the stronger the link becomes and the easier it is to access it

- Mirror exercise to improve self image / set a goal – close eyes and imagine a mirror behind yourself with the image of how you don't want to be, a mirror in front with the way you wish to be – step into the image in front- feel it, notice how good it feels – say something appropriate to yourself, e.g. I'm glad I'm going the right way now' and then open your eyes – repeat several times

- What if? – fears are often less frightening if 'taken out of the bag' and examined . . . take the feared scenario to its worst conclusion – that is only one possibility – what are the others? Are there some positive possibilities? – what would turn a possibility into a probability?

- Stress review time – for people who continually ruminate on their worries – break into the cycle – thought stopping – write down what is worrying you and then do something else – have half an hour a day 'worry time' to look at what you have written and break the worry down if possible – then

  1. Is it your problem?

  2. Can you do anything about it?

  3. Put it in a different time perspective – will it still be important in a year – 10 years – 100 years?

- Three best things – write down the three best things you noticed that day – warmth of a shower, taste or smell of something you ate or drank – something you saw – helps to shift from focus on past/ future to now

- Tomorrow hasn't happened yet – what you do today can start to define tomorrow – set one goal a day – do it and then congratulate yourself – anything else is a bonus – feeling that there is so much you should do and haven't done only feeds feelings of despair/anxiety!

    You can only have one thought at a time – why not make it a good one

    Everest was climbed by placing one foot in front of another
    — but it helps if you have a map

    You are whatever you think you are
    — if you change what you think, then you change what you are

    If you always do what you've always done,
    you'll always get what you've always got!

Insanity is doing the same thing over and over again and expecting a different result.

Worry is interest paid on something that may never happen

Clinical outcome routine evaluation

Therapist:
Client ID: Initial CORE I   ☐
Gender: Final CORE F
Age: Other O. . .

Important – Please Read This First

This form has 34 statements about how you have been OVER THE LAST WEEK.

Please read each statement and think how often you felt that way last week.

Then tick the box which is closest to this

		Not at all	Only occasionally	Sometimes	Often	Most or all the time	OFFICE USE ONLY
1	I have felt terribly alone and isolated	$\square_0$	$\square_1$	$\square_2$	$\square_3$	$\square_4$	$\square_F$
2	I have felt tense, anxious or nervous	$\square_0$	$\square_1$	$\square_2$	$\square_3$	$\square_4$	$\square_P$
3	I have felt I have someone to turn to for support when needed	$\square_4$	$\square_3$	$\square_2$	$\square_1$	$\square_0$	$\square_F$
4	I have felt O.K. about myself	$\square_4$	$\square_3$	$\square_2$	$\square_1$	$\square_0$	$\square_W$
5	I have felt totally lacking in energy and enthusiasm	$\square_0$	$\square_1$	$\square_2$	$\square_3$	$\square_4$	$\square_P$
6	I have been physically violent to others	$\square_0$	$\square_1$	$\square_2$	$\square_3$	$\square_4$	$\square_R$
7	I have felt able to cope when things go wrong	$\square_4$	$\square_3$	$\square_2$	$\square_1$	$\square_0$	$\square_F$
8	I have been troubled by aches, pains or other physical problems	$\square_0$	$\square_1$	$\square_2$	$\square_3$	$\square_4$	$\square_P$
9	I have thought of hurting myself	$\square_0$	$\square_1$	$\square_2$	$\square_3$	$\square_4$	$\square_R$
10	Talking to people has felt too much for me	$\square_0$	$\square_1$	$\square_2$	$\square_3$	$\square_4$	$\square_F$
11	Tension and anxiety have prevented me from doing important things	$\square_0$	$\square_1$	$\square_2$	$\square_3$	$\square_4$	$\square_P$
12	I have been happy with the things I have done	$\square_4$	$\square_3$	$\square_2$	$\square_1$	$\square_0$	$\square_F$
13	I have been disturbed by unwanted thoughts and feelings	$\square_0$	$\square_1$	$\square_2$	$\square_3$	$\square_4$	$\square_P$
14	I have felt like crying	$\square_0$	$\square_1$	$\square_2$	$\square_3$	$\square_4$	$\square_W$
15	I have felt panic or terror	$\square_0$	$\square_1$	$\square_2$	$\square_3$	$\square_4$	$\square_P$
16	I made plans to end my life	$\square_0$	$\square_1$	$\square_2$	$\square_3$	$\square_4$	$\square_R$
17	I have felt overwhelmed by my problems	$\square_0$	$\square_1$	$\square_2$	$\square_3$	$\square_4$	$\square_W$

		Not at all	Only occasionally	Sometimes	Often	Most or all the time	OFFICE USE ONLY
18	I have had difficulty getting to sleep or staying asleep	$\square_0$	$\square_1$	$\square_2$	$\square_3$	$\square_4$	$\square_P$
19	I have felt warmth or affection for someone	$\square_4$	$\square_3$	$\square_2$	$\square_1$	$\square_0$	$\square_F$
20	My problems have been impossible to put to one side	$\square_0$	$\square_1$	$\square_2$	$\square_3$	$\square_4$	$\square_P$
21	I have been able to do most things I needed to	$\square_4$	$\square_3$	$\square_2$	$\square_1$	$\square_0$	$\square_F$
22	I have threatened or intimidated another person	$\square_0$	$\square_1$	$\square_2$	$\square_3$	$\square_4$	$\square_R$
23	I have felt despairing or hopeless	$\square_0$	$\square_1$	$\square_2$	$\square_3$	$\square_4$	$\square_P$
24	I have thought it would be better if I were dead	$\square_0$	$\square_1$	$\square_2$	$\square_3$	$\square_4$	$\square_R$
25	I have felt criticised by other people	$\square_0$	$\square_1$	$\square_2$	$\square_3$	$\square_4$	$\square_F$
26	I have thought I have no friends	$\square_0$	$\square_1$	$\square_2$	$\square_3$	$\square_4$	$\square_F$
27	I have felt unhappy	$\square_0$	$\square_1$	$\square_2$	$\square_3$	$\square_4$	$\square_P$
28	Unwanted images or memories have been distressing me	$\square_0$	$\square_1$	$\square_2$	$\square_3$	$\square_4$	$\square_P$
29	I have been irritable when with other people	$\square_0$	$\square_1$	$\square_2$	$\square_3$	$\square_4$	$\square_F$
30	I have thought I am to blame for my problems and difficulties	$\square_0$	$\square_1$	$\square_2$	$\square_3$	$\square_4$	$\square_P$
31	I have felt optimistic about my future	$\square_4$	$\square_3$	$\square_2$	$\square_1$	$\square_0$	$\square_W$
32	I have achieved the things I wanted to	$\square_4$	$\square_3$	$\square_2$	$\square_1$	$\square_0$	$\square_F$
33	I have felt humiliated or shamed by other people	$\square_0$	$\square_1$	$\square_2$	$\square_3$	$\square_4$	$\square_F$
34	I have hurt myself physically or taken dangerous risks with my health	$\square_0$	$\square_1$	$\square_2$	$\square_3$	$\square_4$	$\square_R$

Creative approaches

When you feel 'stuck'

If a client, or myself, feels stuck I may suggest that we get up and move around. I will also admit to the client that I feel stuck. This nearly always frees things up and allows one's creativity to help. If you start feeling anxious about being stuck it becomes harder to think and act creatively.

Suggesting that the client and I swop chairs and the client (as the therapist) tells me (as the client) what he needs to hear can be useful when stuck. I have been known to pull a client out of their chair and turn them round saying 'Well what would you do with her?' This should only be done when you have good rapport but can act as a useful pattern interrupt.

We have already talked about perceptual positions and sometimes it can be helpful to act these out by having different chairs representing different protagonists or parts of the client such as the younger and older them.

Non-verbal approaches

Sometimes clients have difficulty verbalising their difficulties and here it is very useful to find other methods to help.

I have already talked about writing things down, which I often regard as helpful, and writing letters and poetry are a useful way of helping those so inclined to explore and resolve their feelings. I sometimes suggest that the client might want to imagine themselves in the future when their problems have been resolved and write a letter to me from twelve months in the future telling me what they are doing. This can be helpful in focusing the client on their goals.

Sometimes it can be therapeutic to encourage the client to draw pictures of where the client feels they are now, where they want to be and a third picture of how they might help themselves move from one to the other.

This client actually utilised drawing as her main therapeutic tool. She would draw a picture before each visit and we would then discuss it.

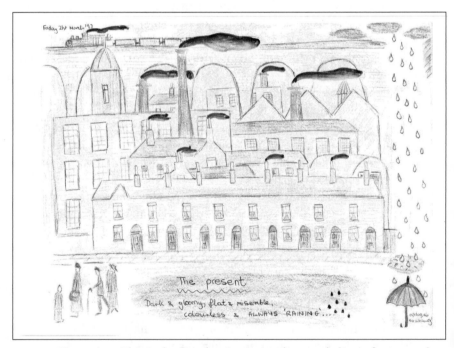

Figure A.1 This is the first drawing a very depressed client of mine made when I asked her to bring me drawings representing where she was, where she wanted to be and a third drawing thinking about how she might make that journey.

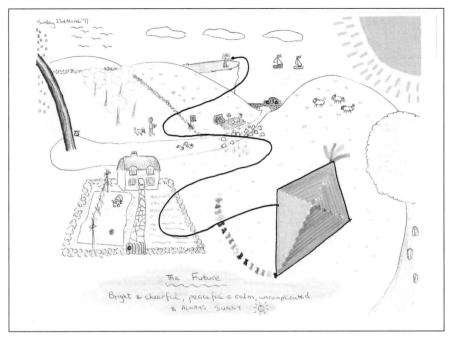

Figure A.2   The second drawing representing where she wanted to be

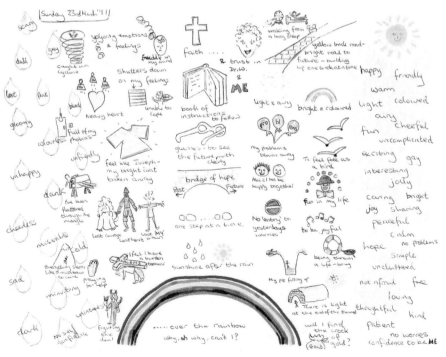

Figure A.3   The third drawing exploring how she might make that journey

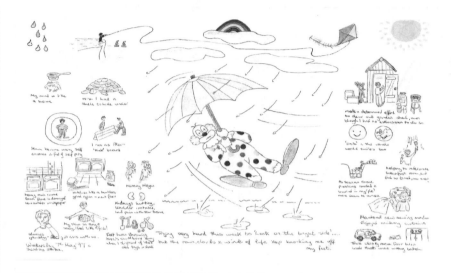

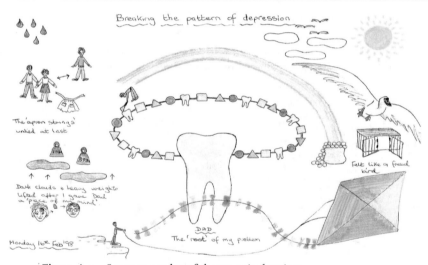

Figure A.4 Some examples of therapeutic drawing

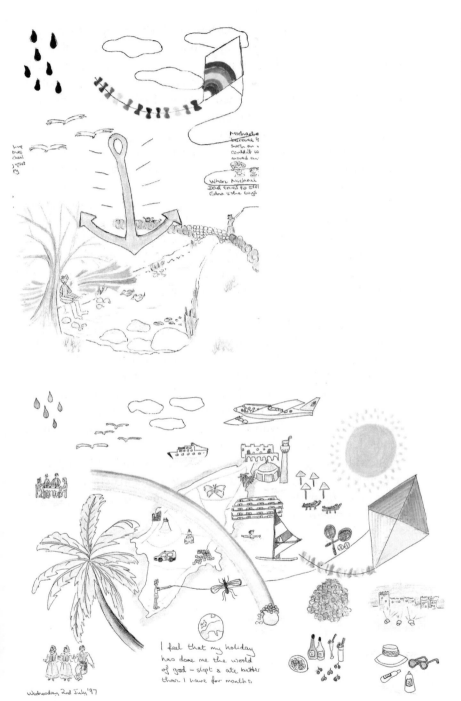

Figure A.4 *Continued*

Drawing can also be used to externalise feelings. In this situation, I suggest that the client uses their non-dominant hand so that they don't feel judgemental about the end results. I ask that they spend five minutes focusing on their emotional distress and just doodle it out on the paper. Then I ask them to take a fresh piece of paper and doodle again while focusing on how they want to be.

Music can also be used in this way. If the client plays an instrument suggesting that they play out their feelings for a few minutes and then play how they want to feel can often be helpful. I have a bodhran (a type of small drum) in my office, which I sometimes offer to clients if they are having difficulty verbalising the problem. They play out the problem on the bodhran and then I ask then to play something that would help. I have a colleague who uses a gong in a similar way.

Working in this way is helping the client to access their unconscious resources as any creative or artistic pursuit accesses 'right brain' processing or our 'unconscious' mind rather than our conscious intellectual rationality.

Movement can also be used effectively. I may suggest that the client pose as a statue depicting how he feels and sees the problem. Then I suggest that he begin to find a movement that would be helpful and explore it. The movement acts as a metaphorical representation of the client's difficulty and encourages them to access internal resources. Gradually, the client changes the movements until he feels that he is connecting with how he wants to be and ends up with a statue that represents his desired state.

As with all the approaches described in this book, it is important to connect the client with how they wish to be and to help them access their inner strengths and resources rather than to continually focus on their problems or difficulties.

Anxiety and depression

Here, I have tabulated the different problems encountered in anxiety and depression and, in bold type, those strategies that can be used to help.

▶ Anxiety

Characterised by:

Adrenalin effects: agitation, lack of concentration, time pressure, fatigue
   Self-hypnosis
   Mindfullness
   Body scan

Negative focus
   Thought stopping
   Pattern interrupts
   Mirror exercise
   Three best things
   Mindfullness

Catastrophisation
   Possibilities and probabilities
   Positive mental rehearsal
   Change internal dialogue

Rumination
Thought stopping
Pattern interrupts
Worry time and the three questions

Feeling overwhelmed and out of control (overactive, flitting)
One small goal at a time
Positive mental rehearsal
Deliberately slow movements down
Take some time out for oneself
3 Ps:- Plan, prioritise and premium time
3 Ds:- Ditch, delegate or do
Learn to say 'No'

▶ **Depression**

Characterised by:

Negative focus
Thought stopping
Pattern interrupts
Mirror exercise
Three best things
Mindfullness

Flatness or hopelessness – pervasiveness
Acknowledge change
Solution orientation
Ego strengthening
Positive suggestion using imagery, e.g. control centre

Personalisation
Perceptual positions
Listening to supportive friend part

Lethargy and lack of motivation/energy
One small goal at a time
Positive mental rehearsal
Mirror exercise

How to apply these ideas in practice – some case studies

Seven 10–15-minute appointments at one-week or two-week intervals and one appointment of 20–30 minutes

David was a 57-year-old mechanic who had been out of work for two years with stress and depression. He came to the surgery frequently with various physical complaints and symptoms and had been on an antidepressant for several months with no noticeable improvement. He said he was reasonably happily married, had two grown up children and felt his own childhood had been unremarkable.

After some discussion he was keen to try a different approach as he was unhappy about taking medication. We decided to have a 10-minute consultation every week for one month and review progress.

Visit 1

Finding out the patterns

Upon asking David how he 'did' anxiety he determined that he first noticed a feeling or a twinge somewhere in his body. This led to catastrophising thoughts (see Chapter 7) such as 'I'm starting to be ill again!' 'I won't be able to . . .' 'Oh God, what's wrong?' which generated more feelings of fear and anxiety . . . and the pattern continued in an ever increasing negative spiral resulting in David withdrawing more and more and suffering increasing levels of anxiety and depression. We also started to look at how his negative focus underpinned his feelings of depression and worthlessness; how his thoughts, behaviour and feelings were all interlinked.

Internal dialogue

I suggested various ways that David might change the impact of these negative thoughts such as changing the voice tone by 'helium-ising' or 'cartoon-ising' the thought, or challenging the thought and deliberately generating alternatives.

Emotional spectacles

I asked David to look around my room and make a mental note of anything that was square or oblong shaped. Having done this, I then asked him how many round objects he had noticed. This demonstrated to him that he only noticed those things that he directed his attention towards. As part of his homework, I asked him to write down every evening in a notebook the three best things he noticed each day, whether these were something he saw, felt, heard, ate or drank.

Mindfullness

I suggested that he could also stop his negative thoughts by deliberately focusing his attention for a few minutes on whatever he was experiencing through his senses; on whatever he could see, hear or smell, without judging it in any way or having any thoughts about it – just being aware of it. If he started to notice other thoughts, he didn't need to follow them but could just take his attention back to noticing what he was sensing at that moment. If he was focused on the present moment he was not agitating about the future or ruminating about the past.

Visit 2

Breathing exercise and the body scan:

I suggested that David get into the habit of taking a few moments now and again to deliberately let go tension on his out breath and allow his muscles to become loose and relaxed. I then took David through the simple breathing exercise detailed in Chapter 10 and suggested ways he could use imagery to get rid of negative thoughts and feelings and replace them with positive ones.

Calmness anchor

When asking David what came to mind when he thought of calmness, peace, and tranquillity, he answered that he thought about being out with his father fishing on the local river. I suggested that he might like to take some time each day to close his eyes, focus on his breathing for a few minutes, throw away any tension or anything else he wanted to be rid of down his rubbish chute and take himself back to that time in his imagination, to connect with those feelings of calmness and enjoyment that could replace what he had thrown away.

Being a detective

I asked David to write down at least three things that he noticed he was thinking and doing differently on days when he felt better and those when he felt not so good, and bring this with him to his next appointment.

Visit 3

Feedback

We looked at the differences between how David behaved and thought on good and not so good days. He identified that on better days he got out of bed in the morning, rather than lying there for an hour or two; he felt better when meeting his friends or talking to them on the phone and he noticed that on better days he had was more able to challenge his negative thought patterns.

Setting goals

He decided that he would get out of bed every morning and have a shower and if he didn't really feel like it he would tell himself that he could always go back to bed afterwards – but he didn't think he actually would. He would also try and talk to a friend every day – even if only on the telephone.

I suggested that he set one specific goal a day; that if he set too many goals he might find that not achieving them all would feed into his negative feeling about himself. I suggested that David write down in his notebook each evening one thing he wanted to do the next day and to feel good when he ticked it off the following evening. Anything else he did that day he could view as a bonus!

David stated that he knew what kind of a day he was going to have as soon as he opened his eyes in the morning, so, to interrupt the thoughts and feeling he was accessing on a not so good day, I suggested that he do the mirror exercise four or five times as soon as he awoke.

Mirror exercise

I suggested that David do the mirror exercise, visualising how he did not want to be in a mirror behind him and then building up the image of how he wanted to be in the mirror in front of him. He then imagined stepping into the image in front, feeling how good it felt and saying something appropriate internally such as 'I know I can do this' and then opening his eyes.

Stressors – worry time and the three questions

I suggested that when he noticed that he was focussing on a particular negative thought or worry (ruminating), that he interrupt himself by moving or counting backwards from 300 in sevens; write the worrying thought down in his notebook and then go and do something else. He was to have a set time each day when he looked at the things he had been worrying about and he was to ask himself three questions.

(1) Is it my problem?

(2) Can I do anything about it? If so, what?

(3) Will it still be important in a year's time?

 In 10 years' time? In a hundred years' time?

Visit 4

Feedback

At the month review, there had been a noticeable improvement and David, when asked how often he felt he needed to attend surgery now, suggested every two weeks.

We decided to meet every two weeks for two months and review.

Changing thoughts and feelings

I asked David to continue to notice his thoughts; to write down some of the more persistent and how they made him feel. I asked him to notice what seemed to 'stress' him and to write this down also. I then asked him to keep a note of what he did to try and help himself on these occasions and whether it worked for him.

Stressful thought or event   Feeling   What did I do?   Did it help?

We decided that he would do this twice a day at least but that if he wanted he could do it on other occasions as well.

Visit 5

Scaling question

David felt that he was at 4.5 out of 10 and said that he needed to work harder at stopping his negative thoughts.

'It's as though I know what I need to do but there's a brick wall in the way'.

Client-generated imagery

The session was spent exploring how he could get around, climb over or in some way get through to the resources he saw as available to himself on the other side of the wall. I asked David to close his eyes and imagine this wall, to describe it to me and then to explore how he might be able to get to the other side. After a while, during which he was obviously processing internally, he decided that he would make the wall into an archway. In this process he was gaining acceptance of the obstacles in his path (the wall) rather than ignoring them (climbing over them) and was using his creativity to utilise the obstacles as a way to progress (making the bricks into an archway).

Visit 6

David reported that he had been feeling much more positive and put himself at 6 out of 10 on the scaling question. He was doing more and had been out for a walk every day so felt he was getting fitter.

Confidence anchor

David had problems with feelings of low confidence and self-esteem, especially since he had been off work and he really enjoyed setting his confidence anchor. He revisited three occasions when he had felt really good about himself – when he had learned to swim, when he had got married, and one time at work when someone he admired had congratulated him on a job well done. He linked these good posi-tive feelings to clenching his right fist and to an internal 'Yeah!' I suggested that he repeat this for himself each time he did his self-hypnosis; allowing his mind to come up with the same or different times when he had felt good and clenching his fist with an internal cheer as he accessed the good feelings. Whenever David felt low he could use his anchor to access good positive feelings.

Visit 7

Criticism and praise

We talked about David's ability to shrug off any praise and how he felt completely devastated by criticism. We talked about the separation of behaviour and identity and how our feelings about ourselves develop (see Chapter 15) as we grow through childhood. I likened praise to a gift that someone gives him and emphasised how criticism is feedback on something we have done . . . and that sometimes it is the critic that has the problem rather than the action being wrong. This led onto . . .

Perceptual positions

We decided we would look at various events that had happened recently; one was an argument with his wife and the other when he had gone into work to see his boss.

I suggested that he stand up and visualise each scenario in turn. I suggested that he run through the event in his imagination and then to do so again after stepping into the 'shoes' of the other person. This would give him insights into how the other person was feeling and how they saw him. He was then to step into an 'Observer' position where he could observe both himself and the other person and their interaction.

David found this very interesting, especially in the work scenario. He realised that he was reacting to his boss with fear as if he was being bullied, which he wasn't in this instance. This led on to a discussion about a previous job where he had been bullied and harassed and left because of it. He realised that he had been 'sensitised' by his past experience and was therefore overreacting.

Visit 8

Feedback

David was progressing well and had reduced his dose of an antidepressant with a view to coming off it within the following month.

Time road metaphor

We talked about how our feelings in the present can be underpinned by similar feelings from the past; that it is as though a younger part of ourselves holds onto those negative feelings to protect us in some way. I suggested that although he could not alter his past, he was greater than the past events that had happened to him and that he could maybe let go negative feelings from the past, once they had served their purpose.

I asked David to close his eyes and imagine his time road with the past in one direction and the future in another. I suggested that he float up above the present and ask his mind to sort out anything relevant from the past and place the events with good feelings attached on one side of the road and those with not such good feelings attached on the other. He could then spend time floating over the good events, connecting with them and gathering up the good feelings from them. He was then to float from his beginnings to the present, high above the not so good events, allowing his unconscious mind to learn what it needed to let the negative feelings go; helping the younger part of himself in any appropriate way to feel comforted, loved and supported, reminding that younger part that however upsetting those times might have been, he survived them, because he was from his future, so he no longer needed to hold onto those negative feelings (see Chapter 16).

David continued to attend every couple of months and maintained his progress. He came off all medication and started back at work; part time at first. He coped well and although he still developed physical symptoms on occasion they were much less of a problem than previously. He continued to use self-hypnosis to keep his stress levels down and recorded his response to the scaling question each week in a notebook. If he noticed that he was beginning to slide down he knew he had strategies that he could use effectively to prevent the downward spiral into depression.

Summary for Case Study 1 – David

Visit 1:
Finding out the patterns
Internal dialogue
Emotional spectacles
Mindfullness

Visit 2:
Breathing exercise and the body scan
Calmness anchor
Being a detective: Thoughts and actions on good and not so good days

Visit 3:
Feedback
Setting goals
Mirror exercise
Stressors – worry time and the three questions

Visit 4:
Feedback
Changing thoughts and feelings
Stressful thought or event   Feeling   What did I do?   Did it help?

Visit 5:
Scaling question
Client-generated imagery

Visit 6:
Confidence anchor

Visit 7:
Criticism and praise
Perceptual positions

Visit 8:
Time road metaphor

Seven 10–15-minute appointments at a week or two-week intervals.

Maureen was a 42-year-old woman who suffered with chronic recurrent depression and low levels of confidence and self-esteem. She had had a disturbed childhood with many moves of location and her parents finally divorcing when she was 13. She rarely saw her father and her mother had died a few years previously. She remarked that they were 'not a very close family'. She had no siblings and had never married. She said she had always felt 'a loner' but had enjoyed her job as a bank teller, although she found it stressful at times. She had several friends but recently had become more withdrawn and depressed following a poor appraisal at work. She had been off work with depression for three months when we met and had been prescribed an antidepressant which she had stopped after a few days because of side effects.

Visit 1

Patterns

Maureen felt that she had first started with depression when she was a child and that she had had recurrences on and off throughout her life usually triggered by a loss such as when her cat had been run over or by extra stress such as appraisals or change in her work circumstances. We talked about how she 'did' depression and how she maintained it over time.

We discussed how patterns of thought, feeling and behaviour could be changed. Maureen also admitted to a great deal of negative, internal and self-critical dialogue. We discussed how she might change the impact of the negative thought by helium-ising or cartoon-ising the voice tone.

I asked her to spend some time over the next week noticing these patterns and maybe having some other ideas of ways she could begin to change them.

Goals

Maureen wanted to feel happier and to be able to get back to work. She wanted to feel more confident and comfortable with herself and when with a group of friends. We talked about motivation and energy. I said that when you are feeling good you get a desire to do something and so you go and do it. When you are depressed you lose that desire and the tendency is to do very little. Doing things without actually wanting to breaks this pattern and the motivation then gradually builds again.

Scaling question

I used the scaling question and asked Maureen to close her eyes and imagine herself one step further up her scale (she was at 1) and to tell me one thing she could do tomorrow that would help her move up to being a 2. She decided that tomorrow she would get up before 9:00 a.m. and have a bubble bath.

I asked her to write down each evening in her notebook the one thing she was going to do the following day to help move herself up the scale and to tick it off and congratulate herself when she had accomplished it. Anything else achieved would be a bonus.

Visit 2

Client-generated metaphor

When asked how she saw her depression Maureen remarked 'It is as though I am in a black hole with no way out'. I asked Maureen to close her eyes and imagine that black hole and to begin to describe what she saw. She described finding a ledge upon she could begin her climb up and then she started to see daylight filtering down into the hole. I suggested that she might like to begin to see how she might climb out and she said that there were many ledges around the walls and maybe she could begin to use them to help herself out. I suggested that she might like to return at various times to see how she was doing and that she would know what to do to help herself and that the most important thing was that she now knew that she could climb out.

Three best things

I asked Maureen to write down each evening the three best things she had noticed during the day.

Focus of attention

I got Maureen to stand with her shoulders hunched and her eyes downcast and feel the difference when she straightened her shoulders and looked upwards.

I then asked her to make a deliberate effort to notice things around her when she went for a walk, to notice the clouds, the chimney pots, (which would encourage her to look upwards) the sounds and the smells. If she was doing this, she would be less inclined to get caught up in negative thoughts.

Visit 3

Utilisation and ego strengthening

I discovered that she was very keen on doing cross-stitch. She had brought in a sample of her work, an elaborate and painstakingly made picture of a rural farm scene. As we looked at it together I asked her to tell me what skills she needed to accomplish this work. Among others we listed persistence, ability to concentrate, attention to detail, dexterity, an eye for colour and a love of beautiful things. This acknowledgement (by her) of some of her strengths was one of her first steps to believing in herself.

Self-hypnosis

I taught Maureen a progressive muscular relaxation and imagery of her special place and I asked her to practise daily for ten minutes or so. She decided to do her self-hypnosis every morning and also in the evening when she went to bed.

Visit 4

Imagery

I took Maureen through the ego strengthening pond and pebbles metaphor (page 113) and suggested that she add this into her regular self-hypnosis.

Playing cards

I took a pack of playing cards – ace high, 2 low and asked Maureen to pick a card that she thought represented her, in this case a 4. I placed this face down on the desk and asked her what card her best friend would give her – a Queen: how would she rate her ability at doing cross-stitch? – a King: how would she rate her ability at cooking? – a Jack: how would she rate her ability at work? – a 10; as a glider pilot? – a 10 . . . each time placing the card chosen on top of the first one. I then picked up the cards she had selected in a pack with the 3 on top saying 'This is what you told me you are' and then fanned out all the other cards saying 'But look at all these you have forgotten about!'

Scaling question

Maureen felt that she was now at about 4 on her scale. She said that what was keeping her from a 3 was telephoning her friend and having a chat each day; she decided that going out for a short walk each day would move her up to a 5.

Visit 5

Feedback

Maureen was feeling much more positive and was talking about a phased return to work.

Negative self-talk and the compassionate friend

Maureen told me that although she wasn't very good at socialising and felt very shy in a group she was a good listener and her friends often seemed to confide in her if they felt troubled. I remarked that she was obviously a good friend and she agreed that if a friend was in trouble she would support and encourage them. I suggested that perhaps she needed to befriend herself and try listening to that compassionate friend part of herself. I suggested that she close her eyes and review a couple of recent situations in which she told me that she had 'beaten herself up' and listen to what that compassionate part of herself had to say. I then got feedback on how that had helped and suggested that she might like to do this every evening until it was something that she would do automatically.

We also looked at the appraisal that had triggered her recent bout of depression and she realised that her appraiser had not been very good at people management and had not been giving constructive criticism. She realised that, although there were instances when she had made mistakes because she had been feeling very stressed, most of the time she had performed adequately and that she had taken the negative feedback too personally, at the level of identity.

Visit 6

Feedback

Maureen was delighted that she was developing the ability to take a step back from her thoughts and feelings, examine and challenge them. She related several instances where she had done this when in the past she would have just listened to her self-criticism and felt bad.

Confidence anchor

Maureen told me that she had gained her glider's license several years ago. She had become quite animated whilst telling me about this and it was obviously a good resource for her, helping her to feel more confident and competent. I asked where she kept the photo of herself standing by the glider that she had described. She replied that it was in a drawer somewhere. I suggested that she find it and hang it somewhere where she would see it and remember and access the good feelings associated with it.

At her next visit she told me that she had hung it in the hall and that she had noticed the good feelings she had each time she looked at it when passing by.

We then set a confidence anchor as described in Chapter 12.

Visit 7

Social confidence and positive mental rehearsal

Maureen was feeling much better but was still apprehensive about being in a group social situation. She was also somewhat apprehensive about her imminent return to work. I suggested that she approach the social situation as a series of one to one conversations (which she was comfortable with). She was due to go on the work's Christmas outing and we did a positive mental rehearsal of the event. She closed her eyes and imagined herself using these strategies and her confidence anchor and talking to her friend later about how much she had enjoyed it when she hadn't really expected to. I suggested that Maureen do a positive mental rehearsal of her return to work and to do an experiment.

Smiling

I suggested that she try smiling at people she met, see what response she got and report back to me at our next session.

Visit 8

Feedback

Maureen's works Christmas 'do' had gone well and she had agreed to meet up with some work colleagues to go and play tenpin bowling after Christmas. She had been surprised at the positive response she had received from the smiling experiment and had noticed that she had felt better as well. We talked about assertiveness and bullying and I showed her how our feelings can be changed by how we picture or represent a person internally to ourselves.

We practised the sub-modality exercise (see page 159) and then devised a 'rescue plan' that she could refer to if she started to feel down.

Maureen's Rescue Plan

Maureen decided that she needed some way of reminding herself of the strategies she could use if she noticed that she was slipping back into a negative state. She decided to make a set of cards that she could put up on her fridge. These were Maureen's cards:-

1. Go for a walk and notice what I see and hear . . . look at the chimney pots!

2. Do 10-minute self-hypnosis and imagery.

3. Do the mirror exercise.

4. Phone a friend.

5. Remember to smile.

6. Write down the three best things each day.

7. Set one small goal a day and do it.

8. Listen to my helpful supportive friend part.

9. Repeat my negative thoughts to myself in a Donald Duck voice.

10. Use my confidence anchor.

11. Write about how I am feeling and then about how I want to feel.

12. Do something, preferably something I enjoy; but do something.

Maureen continued to do well and I saw her from time to time over several years and although she did become depressed on occasion it was never as severe or prolonged and each time she noticed the warning signs she put in place her 'rescue plan' and came out of her depression more quickly.

Summary for Case Study 2 – Maureen

Visit 1:
Patterns
Goals
Scaling question

Visit 2:
Client-generated metaphor
Three best things
Focus of attention

Visit 3:
Utilisation and ego strengthening
Self hypnosis

Visit 4:
Imagery
Playing cards
Scaling question

Visit 5:
Feedback
Negative self-talk and the compassionate friend

Visit 6:
Feedback
Confidence anchor

Visit 7:
Social confidence and positive mental rehearsal
Smiling

Visit 8:
Feedback
Rescue plan

▶ **Case 3: Amy – panic disorder and agarophobia**

> Seven 10–15-minute appointments at one-week or two-week
> intervals and one appointment of 20–30 minutes

Amy, an intelligent 19-year-old, suffered with panic disorder and
agarophobia. She had a supportive family (very necessary if you are
going to be agarophobic) and lived with her mother, father and
younger brother of twelve. She had had a reasonably happy childhood
and, apart from an episode of bullying when she was about nine, she
had enjoyed school. She was a high achiever and was expected to do
very well. She had struggled with examination nerves during her
GCSE years and didn't do as well as expected in her results but had
got a place at the local sixth form college to do her A levels. She had
become increasingly anxious and withdrawn and had had to leave
college after a term and a half. Her first panic attack had occurred
whilst waiting for a bus to go to college and she then also had panic
attacks at college and then later whilst out locally. She had managed
to go out on occasion by car but she had not been out walking from
her house for more than a year. She enjoyed art and drawing and liked
listening to music. She also had a cat whom she loved. When asked
to describe some time when she had felt really good she told me about
a time a couple of years before when she had been on holiday and

gone for a walk along the beach with the wind in her hair and the sun shining. She was obviously able to recall this very vividly.

Visit 1

History

I took her history as detailed above and established that Amy wanted to learn ways of helping herself feel calmer and eventually to be able to go out with her friends and return to her studies. She wanted to do art at university. By directing Amy's attention towards her goals we were moving away from problem based talking.

Revivification

As Amy was able to recall her walk along the seashore so vividly I suggested that she might like to close her eyes and imagine herself back in that time and place and enjoy it. After a couple of minutes I asked her to open her eyes again and tell me whether she had noticed anything changing in her body or her feelings as she did that and she reported feeling more relaxed. I suggested that she might like to use that as a way of relaxing.

Body scan

If ever she became aware of tension in her body she could take a deep breath in and take herself in her imagination to her beach for a few moments, with her eyes either open or closed, and as she breathed out, allow the tension to flow away with the out breath.

Focusing on desired behaviour

I also asked her to write down for me three things that she did differently when she had a day or part of a day when she felt good.

Visit 2

Feedback

I enquired as to what had changed. This question implies that something has indeed changed. Amy reported that she had enjoyed visiting her beach in her imagination and was surprised that she had actually felt quite a bit better, although she had not ventured out. The three things she noticed she did differently when she felt better were texting her bestfriend, getting up earlier and helping her mother prepare the dinner.

Breathing exercise to reduce tension

I taught her the breathing exercise with imagery of her calm place (which she decided was her beach) and the idea of throwing away (down a rubbish chute) anything that she wished to throw away and replacing that with a good feeling represented by a pebble that she could pick up on her beach. I suggested that she practise this each day for ten minutes or so. She decided that the best time to do this exercise would be after breakfast or before bedtime.

Patterns

I asked Amy to tell me how she 'did' anxiety and what actually happened when she started to panic. The first thing she noticed was a feeling in her chest and her heart pounding. She then started to feel nauseous, cold and clammy and as if she were going to pass out.

As with most people with anxiety problems Amy had a lot of internal dialogue with thoughts such as 'I can't do it' 'I'm going to throw up' 'I'm going to faint'.

We talked about the effects of adrenalin and how anxious thoughts trigger adrenalin as much as events. She agreed that she became caught up in a negative spiral that built up until a full blown panic attack occurred.

Pattern interrupts

I suggested various ways that Amy might experiment with to interrupt her panic pattern. She might helium-ise her internal dialogue so that it became funny rather than scary; and we practised helium-ising some of her negative thoughts out loud so that she could register what it would sound like. When she first became aware of the feeling in her chest, instead of thinking 'Oh God, it's happening again!', she might replace that thought with 'I recognise that feeling – it's telling me I'm becoming tense so I need to visit my beach for a few moments'.

She might stop and write down what event had triggered the anxiety and what thoughts and feelings she had had and what she did to help herself and whether it had worked.

Example

Event	Mother late home from work
Feelings	Tightness in chest – anxious
Thoughts	'What's happened?'
	'Maybe she's been in an accident'
	'I'm on my own'

What did I do?	(1) Let go tension on the out breath	**Did it help?**
		Yes
	(2) Think of alternatives	Yes
	(3) Start to watch TV	Yes

She might also start singing a nursery rhyme in her head if she started to feel panicky. Amy decided that 'Ba, Ba, black sheep' was the rhyme she would use.

Mirror exercise

I suggested that Amy do the mirror exercise, visualising how she did not want to be in a mirror behind her and then building up the image of how she wanted to be in the mirror in front of her. She then imagined stepping into the image in front, feeling how good it felt and saying something appropriate internally such as 'I know I can do this' and then opening her eyes. As with many people, Amy had an 'awareness' of how she wanted to be, rather than a clear visual image, but this in no way makes the exercise any less effective. I suggested that she might like to do this exercise every morning before she got out of bed to help her focus on how she wanted to feel.

Visit 3

Feedback

Amy reported feeling generally calmer, she was doing the mirror and the breathing exercises regularly and was finding that going to her beach in her imagination and writing her thoughts down were useful ways of interrupting her panic and anxiety spirals.

Dealing with the past

We discussed how anxiety has a protective value and how the anxiety from the past was probably no longer necessary as she was older and more experienced and had greater strengths and abilities than she had had when she was younger. It is as though that younger part is carrying those feelings of fear for her into the present. Although the events of the past cannot be changed, the feelings attached to them can be. I suggested that her mind knew what that younger her needed in order not to feel anxious and panicky. That that younger her needed to know emotionally what she already knew intellectually - that she wouldn't die in a panic attack – it just felt that way. I suggested that she might like to close her eyes and see that younger her who first felt that anxiety and panic 'Over there' and imagine someone helping her to feel calmer and more able to cope. That someone could be herself from the future, an 'older, wiser her' or some other person that she felt was right. The important thing to do was to comfort and reassure that younger her that however unpleasant the event was, she survived it (because she was from her future) and that she didn't need those feelings of anxiety and fear anymore, once she had learnt what she needed for her protection. She, better than anyone else, knew what that younger part of her needed so as not to feel anxious and afraid.

Having checked with Amy that she had done what needed to be done and that the younger 'her' no longer felt afraid, I suggested that she do the same with any other relevant events her mind brought up for her and then to come back to the here and now, feeling calm and pleased with the work her mind had just done. Amy reported that she had gone back to the time she was bullied and as an adult had told off the bullies and comforted herself. She had also reviewed her first few panic attacks and calmed the younger her, making sure she realised that she hadn't died. She said that she 'felt lighter' and was surprised at how vivid and actually how easy she had found the process.

NB In many cases it is preferable to set up time road imagery as described in David's case but often sufficient dissociation can be obtained by using terminology such as 'Over there'. Be aware that you may need more time for this exercise – I usually schedule a twenty or thirty minute appointment if I am going to use this process. For those with no counselling or psychotherapeutic knowledge it may be advisable not to use this approach but in a more general way to help the client love and reassure the younger part of themselves that was frightened.

Visit 4

Feedback

Amy was continuing to do her breathing exercise and visualisation and writing down and challenging her negative thoughts. She was deliberately making herself become more aware of whatever she was experiencing and finding it easier to take a step back and notice her thoughts and feelings and where they came from.

Anchoring

We talked about how various things could trigger her anxiety feelings and discussed ways that she could use to trigger feelings of confidence. We 'set' a kinaesthetic anchor of pressing the tops of her right index finger and thumb together by suggesting she close her eyes and allow her mind to take her to times when she felt good, in control and confident. She chose her walk on the beach that she had already told me about and also re-experienced the good feelings she had had when her teacher had awarded her a class prize and a time when she had enjoyed a particularly good birthday party with her friends. These latter two events she said had just come into her head and she had not thought about them for ages. This tends to happen when you set up the process by suggesting that they close their eyes and ask their unconscious mind to come up with a really good feeling event from the past rather than having them select it consciously. Clients are often surprised by how much more powerful these memories can be than the ones they might have selected deliberately. This good feeling anchor she could use whenever she felt that she was beginning to feel anxious or out of control.

Experiment

Having taught her some ways of coping with anxiety (breathing, pattern interrupts and a good feeling anchor) we decided she would experiment and see how many lampposts she could walk from home. Once she started to feel anxious she would stop, calm herself, and then retrace her steps.

Visit 5

Feedback

She had surprised herself by finding that she could walk to the end of her road and hadn't really felt very anxious at all.

She had also developed a visual anchor of a blue aura of calmness with which she surrounded herself as she was walking. (When talking about anchors I had mentioned the golden glow seen on the Reddibrek adverts of the time as something that some people liked to imagine as their protection.)

Hierarchy

We made a list of the things she wanted to be able to do, starting with the easiest which was going to the local shop and ending with the hardest which was going up to town on her own so that she could attend college.

Positive mental rehearsal

We took the first item on her list and she closed her eyes, relaxed and then visualised herself coming home after going to the shops and telling her mother how well she had done. She then visualised her trip to the shop, feeling calm and pleased with herself and knowing that if she did start to feel anxious she knew what to do. During these visualisations she was *associated* with her image, not merely seeing herself going through the motions. I suggested that she repeat these visualisations before she actually did it in reality.

Visit 6

Feedback

She was feeling very pleased with herself as she had not only been to the local shop on her own on two occasions but had also been out to Manchester with her parents and had enjoyed the trip. She had also been out to a meal with the family at a restaurant and although she had started to feel a bit panicky she had taken herself to the bathroom and done her breathing, used her anchors and had been able to return to the table and enjoy the rest of the evening.

Change focus

Her next item on the hierarchy was to walk to her friend's house, which was about a mile away. Her friend was very supportive and we decided on another experiment. I suggested that she ring her friend when she was about to set off from her house, at which time her friend would set out to meet her. I suggested that she close her eyes, relax, and allow her imagination to take her on that walk and to visualise where it was that her friend would meet up with her and to notice the specific spot. I then suggested that she would be intrigued to discover whether her imagination was correct or whether they actually met earlier or later. This meant that instead of focussing on possible feelings of anxiety she was focussing on where she would actually meet up with her friend.

Visit 7

Feedback

Amy came in and started telling me about a walk she had had around our local reservoir. She was very proud of herself for having achieved this and she described her walk with great animation and enjoyment.

Anchoring

I had a bowl of pebbles on my window sill and she remarked that some of them were just like a smaller version of the stones she had seen at the water's edge. I suggested that she choose one of my pebbles and let it be a reminder to her of the good time she had had. When she squeezed it in her hand she would be able to step into some of the good feelings that she had associated with her outing. She kept her pebble with her and often used it to remind herself that she could feel calm and confident.

She had not been able to arrange her walk with her friend as her friend had been away but she was planning this for the next week.

Scaling question

I asked where Amy felt she was in relationship to achieving her goals (10) and she reported that she felt she was at 6. I then asked her to let her mind come up with some specific thing she was doing or thinking that was helping her to be at 6 rather than 5, and one specific thing she was doing or thinking that would help her move up to 7.

I suggested that each evening she sit down, close her eyes and do this exercise. I suggested that she keep a record in her notebook so that she could be more aware of how she was progressing. If she noticed she was going down the scale that was also useful information and she could respond to it accordingly.

Positive mental rehearsal

We repeated a positive mental rehearsal on the next couple of steps of her hierarchy, which included going on the train and a bus, firstly with a friend and then on her own.

Visit 8

Feedback

She was delighted with her walk to her friend's house and had indeed met her friend where she thought she would. She had been on the bus and the train with her friend and she had asked her not to actually sit with her and had coped well. She was planning a short bus ride on her own and scored herself at 7 out of 10.

We decided that as she was doing so well we would lengthen the time between her appointments to four weeks. Once she had established a positive feedback loop every accomplishment served to reinforce her feelings of confidence and control.

With further minimal support and encouragement she continued to progress, went to college and later University.

Summary for Case Study 3 – Amy

Visit 1:
History
Revivification
Body scan
Focussing on desired behaviour

Visit 2:
Feedback
Breathing exercise to reduce tension
Patterns and pattern interrupts
Event   Feelings   Thoughts   What did I do?   Did it help?
Mirror exercise

Visit 3:
Feedback
Dealing with the past

Visit 4:
Feedback
Anchoring
Experiment

Visit 5:
Feedback
Hierarchy
Positive mental rehearsal

Visit 6:
Feedback
Change focus

Visit 7:
Feedback
Anchoring
Scaling question
Positive mental rehearsal

Visit 8:
Feedback

Phrases that need challenge or qualification to help your client begin to gain a different perspective

Here are some suggested answers for the exercise on page 78:

Phrase	Challenge with	Challenges
1. 'People scare me'	(c), (g)	(a) What would happen if you did / didn't?
2. 'He makes me feel so angry!'	(e), (g), (i)	(b) Has there ever been a time when you didn't? What was different?
3. 'That was the worst time of all'	(l), (k)	
4. 'I handled that meeting badly'	(c), (g), (h)	(c) In what way?
		(d) Who won't?
5. 'He is better than I am'	(g), (c), (p)	(e) Always . . . all the time . . . every minute of every day?
6. 'I must go to work'	(a)	
7. 'She just makes me feel bad'	(c), (i)	(f) How does it mean that?
8. 'I can't ask her out'	(r), (t), (u)	(g) Why do you feel that?

Phrase	Challenge with	Challenges
9. 'They are out to get me'	(c), (j), (r)	(h) Where is your evidence for that?
10. 'That is not important'	(g), (k)	(i) How does this seem to happen?
11. 'They won't listen to me'	(d), (h)	(j) Who is?
12. 'She hurt me deeply'	(g), (o)	(k) Compared with what?
13. 'I can't fly'	(a), (u)	(l) Worse than what?
14. 'I feel angry'	(e)	(m) What stops you from changing it?
15. 'I can't say no'	(q), (t)	(n) Can you think of any other reasons for someone to do this?
16. 'She's always yelling at me; she hates me'	(f)	(o) How specifically?
17. 'He forgot my birthday; he obviously doesn't really love me'	(f), (n)	(p) Better at/than what?
18. 'I never seem to do anything right'	(g), (h)	(q) Never, ever?
19. 'You can't trust people'	(q), (t), (u)	(r) Who specifically?/Who says?
20. 'I always feel anxious'	(b), (v)	(s) How would she know that?
21. 'I regret my decision'	(m)	(t) Can you think of any time when you can/did?
22. 'If she knew how much I liked him she wouldn't do that'	(g), (h), (s)	(u) What stops you?
23. 'He doesn't like me'	(g), (z)	(v) About what? To whom?
		(z) What leads you to believe that?

▶ **Worksheet 1 – Evaluation of stressors**

STRESSOR [Work/home/leisure]	POSSIBLE ACTION	OBSTACLES?

▶ **Worksheet 2– Exploring thoughts and feelings**

Event	Feelings	Thoughts	What did I do?	Did it help?
Mother late home from work	Tightness in chest Anxious	'What's happened?' 'Maybe she's been in an accident' 'I'm on my own'	(1) Let go tension on the out breath (2) Think of alternatives (3) Start to watch TV	(1) Yes (2) Yes (3) Yes

Catastrophic thought	Possible alternative	Which is more probable?
I might fall out of the aeroplane (A)	I arrive at my destination safely (B)	B
I am going to die (in my panic attack) (A)	My panic attack will subside more quickly if I concentrate on calmness (B)	B

References

Alexander, T.A.F. (1946) *Pyschoanalytic Theory*. New York: Ronald Press.

Alloy, L.B. & Abramson, L.Y. (1979) Judgement of contingency in depressed and nondepressed students: Sadder but wiser? *Journal of Experimental Psychology: General*, 108, 441–485.

Andreas, S. & Andreas, C. (1987) *Change your Mind – and Keep the Change*, Moab, UT: Real People Press.

Arkowitz, H. (1997) Clients as cognitive therapists for their own depression. *Convention of the Society for the Exploration of Psychotherapy Integration*, Toronto, Canada.

Asen, E., Tomson, D., Young, V. & Tomson, P. (2004) *Ten Minutes for the Family – Systemic Interventions in Primary Care*. London and New York: Routledge.

Assay, T.P. & Lambert, M.J. (1999) The empirical case for the common factors in therapy: Quantitative findings. In M.A. Hubble, B.L. Duncan & S.D. Miller (eds) *The Heart and Soul of Change: What Works in Therapy*. Washingon, DC: APA Press.

Balint, M. (1957) *The Doctor, His Patient and The Illness*, Edinburgh: Churchill Livingstone.

Bandler, R. & Grinder, J. (1981) *Tranceformations: Neurolinguistic Programming and the Structure of Hypnosis*. Boulder, CO: Real People Press.

Beaulieu, D. (2006) *Impact Techniques for Therapists*. New York and London: Routledge.

Beck, A. T. (1976) *Cognitive Therapy and Emotional Disorders*, New York, International Universities Press.

Beutler, L. & Clarkin, J. (1990) *Systematic Treatment Selection: Toward Targeted Therapeutic Interventions*. New York: Brunner-Mazel.

Beutler, L.E. (1998) Identifying empirically supported treatments: what if we didn't? *Journal of Consulting and Clinical Psychology*, 66, 113–120.

Blatt, S.J., Stanislow, C.A., Zuroff, D.C. & Pilkonis, P.A. (1996) Characteristics of effective therapists: Further analyses of the National Institute of Mental Health Treatment of Depression Collaborative Research Programme. *Journal of Consulting and Clinical Psychology*, 64, 162–171.

Boeree, D.C.G. (2000) *The History of Psychology*. [Electronic publication] http://webspace.ship.edu/cgboer/historyofpsych/html.

Castonguay, L.G., Goldfried, M.R., Wiser, S., Raue, P. & Hayes, A.M. (1996) Predicting the effect of cognitive therapy for depression: A study of unique and common factors. *Journal of Consulting and Clinical Psychology*, 64, 497–504.

Danesi, M. (1989) The neurological coordinates of metaphor. *Communication and Cognition*, 22(1), 73–86.

Danton, W.G. & Antonuccio, D.O. (1997) A focused empirical analysis of treatments for panic and anxiety. In S. Fisher & R.P. Greenberg (eds) *From Placebo to Panacea: Putting Psychiatric Drugs to the Test*. New York: Wiley.

Deitchman, W.S. (1980) How many case managers does it take to screw in a light bulb? *Hospital and Community Psychiatry*, 31, 788–789.

Diagnostic and Statistical Manual of Mental Disorders (DSM IV) (1994). Arlington, VA: American Psychiatric Association.

Duncan, B.L. & Miller, S.D. (2000) *The Heroic Client: Doing Client-Directed, Outcome Informed Therapy*. San Fransico: Jossey-Bass, Inc.

Edwards, B. (1993) *Drawing from the Right Side of the Brain*. London: Harper Collins.

Elder, A. & Holmes, J. (2002) *Mental Health in Primary Care – A New Approach*. Oxford: Oxford University Press.

Elkin, I., Shea, T., Watkins, J.T., Imber, S.D., Sotsky, S.M., Collins, J.F., Glass, D.R., Pilkonis, P.A., Leber, W.R., Docherty, J.P., Fiester, S.J. & Parloff, M.B. (1989) National Institute of Mental Health Treatment of Depression Collaborative Research Programme: General effectiveness of treatments. *Archives of General Psychiatry*, 46, 971–982.

Ellis, A. (1962) *Reason and Emotion in Psychotherapy*. Secausus, NJ: Lyle Stuart.

Ellis, A. (1973) *Humanistic Psychotherapy: The Rational-Emotive Approach*, New York: McGraw-Hill.

Ellis, A. (1989) Rational-Emotive Therapy. In R. Corsini (ed.) *Current Psychotherapies*, Itasca, IL: F.E. Peacock.

Erickson, M.H. (1980) The use of symptoms as an integral part of hypnotherapy. In E. Rossi (ed.) *The Collected Papers of Milton H. Erickson on Hypnosis*. New York: Irvington.

Erickson, M.H. & Rossi, E.I. (1979) *Hypnotherapy: An Exploratory Case-Book*. New York: Irvington.

Eron, J. & Lund, T. (1996) *Narrative Solutions in Brief Therapy*. New York: Guilford.

Evans, C., Mellor-Clark, J., Margison, F., Barkham, M., Mcgrath, G., Connell, J. & Audin, K. (2000) Clinical Outcomes in Routine Evaluation: The CORE-OM. *Journal of Mental Health*, 9, 247–255.

Eysenk, H.J. (1976) The learning theory model of neurosis: a new approach. *Behaviour Research and Therapy*, 14, 251–267.

Flammer, E. & Bongartz, P.W. (2003) On the efficacy of hypnosis: a meta-analytic study. *Contemporary Hypnosis*, 20(4), 179–197.

Freud, S. (1923 / 1960) *The Ego and the Id*. New York: W W Norton.

Gingerich, W.J. & Eisengart, S. (2000) Solution-focused brief therapy: a review of the outcome research. *Family Process* 39(4), 477–498.

Goldberg, D. & Huxley, P. (1992) *Common Mental Disorders, a bio-social model*. Routledge.

Greenberg, R.P., Bornstein, R.F., Greenberg, M.D. and Fisher, S. (1992) A meta-analysis of antidepressant outcome under 'blinder' conditions. *Journal of Consulting and Clinical Psychology*, 60, 664–669.

Greenberg, R.P., Bornstein, R.F., Zborowski, M., Fisher, S. & Greenberg, M.D. (1994) A meta-analysis of fluoxetine outcome in the treatment of depression. *Journal of Nervous and Mental Disease*, 182, 547–551.

Health and Safety Executive (2005) *Stress-related and Psychological Disorder.* London: HSE.

Henry, W., Strupp, H., Butler, S., Schacht, T. & Binder, J. (1993) Effects of training in time-limited dynamic psychotherapy: changes in therapist behaviour. *Journal of Consulting and Clinical Psychology*, 61, 434–440.

Hodgkinson, P.E. (1980) Treating abnormal grief in the bereaved. *Nursing Times*, 17 January.

Hubble, M.A., Duncan, B.L. & Miller, S.D. (1999) Directing attention to what works. In M.A., Hubble, B.L. Duncan & S.D. Miller (eds) *The Heart and Soul of Change: What Works in Therapy.* Washington, DC: APA Press.

Joffe, R., Sokolov, S. & Streiner, D. (1996) Antidepressant treatment of depression: a meta-analysis. *Canadian Journal of Psychiatry*, 41, 613–616.

Kane S, O.K. (Ed.) (2004) *The Art of Therapeutic Communication; The Collected Works of Kay F Thompson.* Carmarthen, Wales: Crown House Publishing Ltd.

Kirsch, I., Montgomery, G. & Sapirstein, G. (1995) Hypnosis as an adjunct to cognitive-behavioural psychotherapy: a meta-analysis. *Journal of Consulting and Clinical Psychology*, 63, 214–220.

Kirsch, I. & Sapirstein, G. (1998) Listening to Prozac but hearing placebo: a meta-analysis of antidepressant medication. *Prevention and Treatment.* www.journals.apa.org/prevention/volume1/pre0010002ahtml

Klerman, G. (1988) Overview of the cross-national collaborative panic study. *Archives of General Psychiatry*, 45, 407–412.

Kopp, R.R. (1995) *Metaphor Therapy – Using Client-Generated Metaphor in Psychotherapy.* New York: Brunner/Mazel Inc.

Lambert, M.J. (1992) Implications of outcome research for psychotherapy integration. In J.C. Norcross & M.R. Goldfried (eds) *Handbook of Psychotherapy Integration.* New York: Basic Books.

Langer, S. (1942/1979) *Philosophy in a New Key: A Study in the Symbolism of Reason, Rite and Art.* Cambridge, MA: Harvard University Press.

Lebovits A H, Twersky, R. & McEwan, B. (1999) Intraoperative therapeutic suggestions in day-case surgery: are there benefits for postoperative outcome? *British Journal of Anaesthesia*, 82(6), 861–866.

Levi-Agresti J. (1968) Differential perceptual capacities in major and minor hemispheres. *Proceedings of the National Academy of Sciences*, 61, 1151.

Lindemann, E. (1944) Symptomatology and management of acute grief. *American Journal of Psychiatry*, 27(4), 593–610.

Madigan, S. & Epston, D. (1995) From 'spy-chiatric gaze' to communities of concern: from professional monlogue to dialogue. In S. Friedman (ed.) *The Reflecting Team in Action: Collaborative Practice in Family Therapy.* New York: The Guilford Press.

McDermott, I. & O'Connor, J. (1996) *NLP and Health.* London: Thorsons.

Mehrabian, A. (1971) *Silent Witness*, Belmont, CA: Wadsworth.

Meichenbaum, D. (1977) *Cognitive-Behaviour Modification: An Integrative Approach*, New York, Plenum.

Mellor-Clark, J., Barkham, M., Connell, J. & Evans, C. (1999) Practice-based evidence and need for a standardised evaluation system: informing the design of the CORE System. *European Journal of Psychotherapy, Counselling and Health*, 2, 357–374.

Miller, A. (1986) *Imagery in Scientific Thought: Creating 20th-Century Physics*. Cambridge MA: The MIT Press.

Montgomery, G.H., Duhamel, K. & Redd, W.H. (2000). A meta-analysis of hypnotically induced analgesia: how effective is hypnosis? *International Journal of Clinical and Experimental Hypnosis*, 48(2), 138–153.

Montgomery, G.H., David, D, Winkel, G., Silverstein, J.H. & Bovbjerg, D.H. (2002) The effectiveness of adjunctive hypnosis with surgical patients: a meta-analysis. *Anaesthesia and Analgesia*, 94, 1639–1645.

Montgomery G.H., Weltz, C.R., Seltz, M., & Bovbjerg, D.H. (2002) Brief presurgery hypnosis reduces distress and pain in excisional breast biopsy patients. *The International Journal of Clinical and Experimental Hypnosis*, 50(1), 17–32.

Murray, E. & Jacobson, L. (1978) Cognition and learning in traditional and behavioural therapy. In S. Garfield, & A. Bergen, (eds.) *Handbook of Psychotherapy and Behaviour Change*, New York, Wiley.

Office of National Statistics (2000) Psychiatric morbidity among adults living in private households in Great Britain. London: Office of National Statistics.

Office of National Statistics (2001) Better or worse: a longitudinal study of the mental health of adults living in private households in Great Britain. London: Office of National Statistics.

Office of National Statistics (2005) Prescriptions dispensed in the community, statistics for 1994–2004. *England, Bulletin 2005*, 02/HSCIC, ONS and NHS.

O'Hanlon, W.H. & Martin, M. (1992) *Solution-Oriented Hypnosis – An Ericksonian Approach*, New York and London: W W Norton & Company, Inc.

Orlinsky, D.E., Grawe, K. & Park, B.K. (1994) Process and outcome in psychotherapy. In A.E. Bergin & S.L. Erfield (eds) *Handbook of Psychotherapy and Behaviour Change*, 4th edn. New York: Wiley.

Patton, M. & Meara, M. (1982) The analysis of language in psychological treatment. In R. Russell, R. (ed.) *Spoken Interaction in Psychotherapy*. New York: Irvington.

Prescription Pricing Authority (2005) Drugs used in mental health—prescribing review. www.ppa.org.uk

Rapp, C.A. & Goscha, R.J. (2006) *The Strengths Model: Case Management with People with Psychiatric Disabilities*. New York: Oxford University Press, Inc.

Ricoeur, P. (1979) The metaphorical process. In S. SACKS (ed.) *On Metaphor*. Chicago: University of Chicago Press.

Rosenthal, R. & Rubin, D.B. (1978) Interpersonal expectancy effects: The first 345 studies. *Behavioural and Brain Sciences*, 3, 377–386.

Rossi E.L., Cheek D.B. (1994) *Mind-Body Therapy; Methods of Ideodynamic Healing in Hypnosis*. New York: W W Norton & Company, Inc.

The Sainsburg Centre for Mental Health and the Northern Ireland Association for Mental Health (2004) Counting the cost. http://www.scmh.org.uk/8025694D00337EF1/vWeb/fsCPIR4PDJ8T

Schon, D. (1983) *The Reflective Practitioner*. London: Temple Smith.

Seligman, M.E.P. (1995) The effectiveness of psychotherapy: The Consumer Reports Survey. *American Psychologist*, 50, 965–974.

Sellick, S.M. & Zaza, C. (1998) Critical review of five nonpharmacologic strategies for managing cancer pain. *Cancer Prevention and Control*, 2(1), 7–14.

Shazer, S.D. (1988) *Clues: Investigating Solutions in Brief Therapy*. New York: W W Norton.

Shazer, S.D. (1994) Essential, non-essential: Vive la difference. In J.K. Zeig (ed.) *Ericksonian Methods: The Essence of the Story*. New York: Brunner-Mazel.

Shazer, S. D. (2005) *More than Miracles: The State of the Art of Solution-Focused Therapy*, Binghampton, NY: Haworth Press.

Shazer, S.D., Berg, I., Lipchik, E., Nunnally, E., Molnar, A., Gingerich, W. & Weiner-Davis, M. (1986) Brief therapy: focused solution development. *Family Process*, 25, 207–222.

Shea, M., Elkin, I., Imber, S., Sotsky, S., Watkins, J., Collins, J., Pilkonis, P., Beckham, R., Glass, D., Dolan, C. & Parloff, M. (1992) Course of depressive symptoms over follow-up: findings from the National Institute of Mental Health Treatment of Depression Collaborative Research Programme. *Archives of General Psychiatry*, 49, 782–787.

Skinner, B. F. (1953) *Science and Human Behaviour*, New York, Macmillan.

Strupp, H. (1996) The Tripartite model and the Consumer Reports Study. *American Psychologist*, 51, 1017–1024.

Syrjala, K.L., Cummings, C. & Donaldson, G.W. (1992) Hypnosis or cognitive behavioral training for the reduction of pain and nausea during cancer treatment: a controlled clinical trial. *Pain*, 48, 137–146.

Tallman, K. & Bohart, A. (1999) The client as a common factor: clients as selfhealers. In M. Hubble, B. Duncan & S. Miller (eds) *The Heart and Soul of Change: What Works in Therapy*. Washington, DC: APA Press.

Thomas, N. (2005) Mental imagery. In E.N.Zalta (ed.) *The Stanford Encyclopedia of Philosophy*. http://plato.Stanford.edu/archives/fall2005/entries/mental-imagery/

Valstein, E. (1998) *Blaming the Brain*. New York: Free Press.

Verbrugge, R.R. & McCarrel, W.S. (1977) Metaphoric comprehension: studies in reminding and resembling. *Cognitive Psychology*, 9, 494–533.

Walters, J. & Peller, J. (2000) *Recreating Brief Therapy: From Preferences to Possibilities*. New York: Norton.

Wampold, B.E., Mondin, G.W., Moody, M., Stich, F., Benson, K. & Ahn, H. (1997) A meta-analysis of outcome studies comparing bone fide psychotherapies: empirically 'All Must Have Prizes'. *Psychological Bulletin*, 122, 203–215.

Watzlawick, P., Weakland, J. & Fisch, R. (1974) *Change: Problem Formation and Problem Resolution*. New York: Norton.

Wexler, B. & Cicchetti, D. (1992) The outpatient treatment of depression: implications of outcome research for clinical practice. *Journal of Mental and Nervous Disease*, 180, 277–286.

Winner, E. (1988) *The Point of Words: Children's Understanding of Metaphor and Irony.* Cambridge, MA: Harvard University Press.

Winnicott, D.W. (1958) *Through Paediatrics to Psycho-Analysis.* London: Hogarth Press.

Wolpe, J. (1958) *Psychotherapy by Reciprocal Inhibition.* Stanford, CA: Stanford University Press.

Young-Eisendrath, P. & Hall, J. (1991) *Jung's Self Psychology: A Constructivist Perspective.* New York: The Guilford Press.

Index